U.S.-
BO
HEALTH

Dedicated to our parents

Sheila and Richard Power
Sylvia and Bryce Byrd

U.S.-MEXICO BORDER HEALTH

Issues for Regional and Migrant Populations

J. Gerard Power
Theresa Byrd

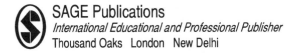
SAGE Publications
International Educational and Professional Publisher
Thousand Oaks   London   New Delhi

For information:

SAGE Publications, Inc.
2455 Teller Road
Thousand Oaks, California 91320
E-mail: order@sagepub.com

SAGE Publications Ltd.
6 Bonhill Street
London EC2A 4PU
United Kingdom

SAGE Publications India Pvt. Ltd.
M-32 Market
Greater Kailash I
New Delhi 110 048 India

Printed in the United States of America

Library of Congress Cataloging-in-Publication Data

Main entry under title:

US-Mexico border health: Issues for regional and migrant
populations / edited by J. Gerard Power and Theresa Byrd.
        p. cm.
    Includes bibliographical references and index.
    ISBN 0-7619-0895-1 (acid-free paper)
    ISBN 0-7619-0896-X (pbk.: acid-free paper)
    1. Public health—Mexican-American Border Region.
    I. Power, J. Gerard. II. Byrd, Theresa.
    RA446.5.M49 U8 1998
    362.1'09721—ddc21   98-8903

This book is printed on acid-free paper.

98 99 00 01 02 03 10 9 8 7 6 5 4 3 2 1

Acquiring Editor:	Dan Ruth
Editorial Assistant:	Anna Howland
Production Editor:	Sanford Robinson
Production Assistant:	Denise Santoyo
Book Designer/Typesetter:	Marion Warren
Indexer:	Teri Greenberg
Print Buyer:	Anna Chin

CONTENTS

ACKNOWLEDGMENTS

We would like to express our thanks to several people who, in various ways, have helped to bring this book to completion. Susan Navarro, Moraima Salazar, Andrea Steege, Carla Cardoza, and Martín Armendariz assisted in the logistics of correspondence between the editors and the contributors. Bruce Neville of the University of Texas at El Paso library and Becky Zima of the Texas Department of Health were extremely helpful in locating reference materials and health statistics. Daniel Ruth of Sage Publications has been very supportive of the project, and the book has benefited from his suggestions. Sharon Thompson saved us by taking care of formatting and editing details. Moral support was provided in plenty by Dr. Connie Della-Piana, Samuel Reveles, Sheila and Richard Power, and Bryce and Sylvia Byrd. Our contributors were extremely patient in the revisions of their manuscripts and in their prompt return.

Finally, we are grateful to the people of the U.S.-Mexico border who were interviewed, studied, examined, analyzed, and described. Their cooperation made this work a reality.

＄

INTRODUCTION

J. GERARD POWER
THERESA BYRD

From the Gulf of Mexico to the Pacific Ocean, the border that divides and joins Mexico and the United States of America stretches for nearly 2,000 miles. The four states on the U.S. side are California, Arizona, Texas, and New Mexico, and the six states on the Mexico side are Baja California, Sonora, Chihuahua, Coahuila, Nuevo León, and Tamaulipas (see map, Appendix A). The Rio Grande, called the Rio Bravo in Mexico, starting at the sister cities of El Paso, Texas, and Ciudad Juárez, Chihuahua, and continuing to Brownsville, Texas, and Matamoros, Tamaulipas, defines about 1,200 miles of the border. There is no natural boundary from San Diego, California, and Tijuana, Baja California, to El Paso and Ciudad Juárez, "only an imaginary line agreed on by the governments of both countries" (Suárez y Toriello & Chávez, 1996, p. 9). The border area contains 107 villages, towns, and cities on the north side and 302 on the south side, with a population of approximately 10 million people living in the 250,000-square-mile border area (El Paso Community Foundation, 1996).

The U.S.-Mexico border presents a unique set of challenges to professionals and lay workers interested in health education and promotion. This uniqueness derives not only from its geographic location and largely arid topography but also from the socioeconomic conditions and the ethnic, linguistic, and cultural demographics of its population. One interesting characteristic of the U.S.-Mexico border is the enormous population movement that takes place on a daily basis. In the El Paso/Juárez area in 1993, there were over 61 million legal crossings from south to north (University of Texas System, 1994). This movement takes place because of the interconnectedness of the people on the border. They cross to work, to shop, and to visit family and friends. Because of this constant flow back and forth across the border, and because of the proximity of the sister cities, it is impossible to characterize any health problem as "belonging" to one country or the other. In this region, it becomes clear that health, safety, environmental, and social issues know no borders.

Second, border communities have experienced a rapid growth in population over the last 20 years. This has given rise to an overwhelming demand on the physical environment and on public services. Between 1980 and 1990, the national population increase for all of Mexico was 21.5%, while growth on the border was 33.9%. In the United States during that time period, the national rate of growth was 10%, while on the border the rate of growth was 31% (University of Texas System, 1994). Migration to the region accounts for about half of the total population growth along the border (Ham-Chande & Weeks, 1992). Much of this migration to the border can be attributed to the growth of the *maquiladora* industry over the last 20 years. *Maquiladoras,* or "twin plants," are production and assembly operations, most often owned by U.S. companies and located in Mexico, where large numbers of semiskilled and unskilled laborers are hired. As of 1986, there were 806 twin plants located in the Mexican border states of Sonora, Baja California Norte, Chihuahua, Coahuila, and Tamaulipas (Stoddard, 1987). By 1996, there were 1,572 in these same states (A. Jimenez, personal communication, September 1996).

Third, an outcome of the population growth in the border region has been the development of substandard residential subdivisions on both sides of the border that lack basic amenities such as water, wastewater services, and paved roads. These subdivisions are referred to as *colonias,* which in Mexican Spanish usually means a neighborhood. In the border context, *colonia* is used to describe an area of extreme poverty lacking an adequate infrastructure. Residents are often exposed to waterborne bacteria and toxic substances such as lead. In addition, these subdivisions are not subject to zoning regulations and consequently have nonstandard and unsafe electrical wiring, plumbing, and construction. It is estimated that over 390,000 people live in Texas *colonias* and that over 42,000 live in New Mexico *colonias* (Environmental Protection Agency, 1996). These substandard residential areas are not as prevalent in Arizona or in California. *Colonias* serve as breeding grounds for disease and illness. The lack of clean water and the sanitation problems that plague these neighborhoods give rise to dysentery, hepatitis A (three times the U.S. national average), typhus, cholera, and tuberculosis (University of Texas System, 1994).

Fourth, water supplies for drinking and bathing are often not available or are threatened by the lack of adequate sewage treatment facilities in many border communities. On the Mexican side of the border, only 88% of the population have access to drinking water, and 69% have access to sewage systems (Environmental Protection Agency, 1996). The most polluted river in the United States is the New River, which flows across the border near Calexico, California. It is estimated that the river carries more than 280 million gallons a day of industrial waste and sewage. The viruses identified in the New River include polio, cholera, typhoid, and hepatitis. The Rio Grande, which divides Texas from its Mexican neighbors, is also one of the most polluted rivers in the United States. The pollution comes from two sources: untreated sewage discharged daily on the Mexican side and the disposal of toxic wastes by *maquiladoras*. In the cities along the border, the health of residents is also threatened by poor air quality. Air pollutants of concern include ozone, particulate matter, carbon monoxide, and sulfur dioxide (Environmental Protection Agency, 1996).

Fifth, many border residents work as migrant or seasonal farm laborers and suffer from a lack of access to health care resources (Bollini & Siem, 1996; Hibbeln, 1996). In Texas, 74% of the entire migrant and seasonal farmworker population lives on the border, and 22% of persons living in the border counties are migrant or seasonal farmworkers (University of Texas System, 1994). From late spring to early fall each year, these farmworkers from the Rio Grande area travel to other states, including California, Oregon, Florida, and Michigan, and return to the region late each fall. Health problems can be spread beyond the border as migrant workers and regional produce make their way northward. For example, contaminated cantaloupes from farms in the Rio Grande valley of Texas were blamed for the 1991 outbreak of salmonella in 23 U.S. states and in Canada. In 1990, the measles epidemic in Washington traced 26% of the cases to Mexico. The malaria epidemic in Florida from 1988 to 1990 was a result of infected Mexican and Central American migrant farmworkers' being bitten by local mosquitoes, which then carried the infection to other residents of the area (Hearn, 1993).

Finally, the demographic profile of the border region also presents some unique health care problems. The population is primarily Hispanic, Spanish speaking, and poor. In the *colonias,* 97.3% of the residents are Hispanic. About two thirds were born in the United States, and approximately 37% have no proficiency in spoken English. These characteristics, as well as the high value placed on family and religion, give rise to some unique challenges in terms of language use and cultural patterns that influence health behavior (Castillo, 1996). The wide disparity between the haves and the have-nots in Mexico has also contributed to unusual health practices in the border region among poor and wealthy Mexicans. Motivated partly by the health services available on the U.S. side as well as the citizenship-by-birth laws in the United States, many poor pregnant Mexican women have crossed the border to give birth on the U.S. side. This practice was much more common before the implementation of the U.S. border patrol strategies (Operation Blockade and Operation Hold the Line) to reduce the number of undocumented immigrants entering the United States from Mexico (Guendalman & Jasis, 1992). On the other end of the continuum, for-profit U.S. hospitals and health service organizations have been soliciting business from wealthy Mexican nationals in the border region. These U.S. businesses have already conducted market research studies to identify their potential client base on the Mexican side of the border (Castillo, 1996). Another unique characteristic of the border population is the high rate of diabetes among Hispanics. Diabetes has a much higher prevalence among Hispanics in general and Mexican Americans in particular than in the general population (Brown & Hanis, 1995; Elshaw, Young, Saunders, McGurn, & Lopez, 1994; Hibbeln, 1996). In the migrant family, diabetes is 338% above the U.S. average (Dever, 1991).

Building on the uniqueness of this region but also recognizing how much can be learned about health promotion and education from border experiences, this book has four primary objectives: first, to highlight the importance of cultural values and behavior patterns that influence health campaigns and health education efforts aimed at migrant farmworker, Mexican, Mexican American, Spanish-speaking, and border populations; second, to identify the challenges to health educators and practitioners working in border regions where the target groups have access to two very different health systems; third, to propose recommendations and models for health promotion that have been tested among border populations; and fourth, to emphasize the centrality of community in health promotion efforts that target groups living in the U.S.-Mexico border region. Although the chapters in this book focus specifically on one region, many of the insights, recommendations, and research findings have implications for health education and promotion in multiple national and international contexts. This book is a compilation of research studies and practitioner reports on a broad range of health concerns facing the population of the U.S.-Mexico border region. Though it is divided into four thematic sections, the themes addressed by many of the chapters in each section overlap. The contributors in Part 1 examine how the cultural values of the border population influence their responses to health messages and their willingness to participate in health programs. Murphy (Chapter 1) focuses on the miscommunications and misunderstandings arising from the interactions between individuals and systems rooted in Mexican collectivist and U.S. individualist value orientations. She draws on two studies to illustrate how these differences affect end-of-life decision making and choices about safer sexual practices among Hispanics and non-Hispanics. In a similar vein, Hinojosa (Chapter 2) reports on a dramatic increase in organ donations among Hispanics in the border region resulting from the change in cultural sensitivity and bilingual skills of the organ bank staff. Using examples from her experiences, she identifies a range of challenges to organ donation among Hispanics and the strategies she has employed to address them. Recognizing the unique set of factors that facilitate the consumption of both legal and illegal drugs in the border region, Lawrence (Chapter 3) compares data from a sample of non-Hispanic whites and Mexican Americans. She documents the different relationships between psychological risk factors and substance abuse in these two groups living in a border town. Finally, in their evaluation of hantavirus education materials designed by the Centers for Disease Control, Crabtree and Ford (Chapter 4) describe the challenges to health communicators working in the border region. Focusing specifically on research conducted among migrant farmworkers, the authors identify a range of obstacles, including language, literacy, access to research participants, and the involvement of multiple bureaucracies.

Part 2 addresses a range of health issues that are complicated by the close proximity of two very different cultures and health systems. Power (Chapter 5) examines alcohol and tobacco advertising in the border region. Because of the proximity to Mexico, border populations are exposed to alcohol and tobacco advertising that is less strictly regulated than in the United States. This set of circumstances gives rise to a unique situation for health promotion, particularly among Spanish-speaking populations living along the border. Identifying the characteristics of health services on both sides of the U.S.-Mexico border, Hopewell (Chapter 6) documents the possibilities for cross-border cooperation in binational tuberculosis control. She describes two different binational efforts in Laredo/Nuevo Laredo and El Paso/Ciudad Juárez. Ramirez-Valles, Zimmerman, Suarez, and De la Rosa (Chapter 7) describe and substantiate how HIV/AIDS prevention programs are complicated in the border region because of the ease with which border populations can cross back and forth. These complications are illustrated in their description of a community-based education project among gay men conducted in the border city of Ciudad Juárez. Ease of movement across the border is also central to the research described by Parietti, Ferreira-Pinto, and Byrd (Chapter 8). They provide evidence of the consumption of unprescribed contraceptives purchased by female adolescents from the United States in Mexican pharmacies across the border.

Part 3 brings together three models of health promotion that have been adopted in the border context. Ford, Barnes, Crabtree, and Fairbanks (Chapter 9) discuss the multiple roles of female community-based health advisors (*promotoras*) in the border region from a public health and a communication perspective. They highlight the function of these women as role models for health promotion efforts in the social networks in which they operate. Schlesinger (Chapter 10) describes the history, current successes, and future plans of Project Vida, a multiple-social-service agency serving a border population, characterizing it as a "model that works." A key component of the success of Project Vida is its community-based programs staffed by community volunteers and employees—a model that could be replicated at other sites. Ramos, Ferreira-Pinto, and Ramos (Chapter 11) compare two case studies of adolescent drug use interventions targeted to young Mexican males. Although building on existing programs in the United States, these models are rather innovative in this population.

Part 4 focuses on the centrality of community in health promotion efforts on the border. Drawing on her expertise as a public health practitioner and as a researcher, Byrd (Chapter 12) reviews the range of community-based programs that are advocated in the literature and evaluates how they are adopted in the border context. She focuses specifically on Project Verdad, a program with which she worked in Ciudad Juárez for a number of years. Lara (Chapter 13) focuses on the challenges to health outreach programs in *colonia* communities on the U.S.-Mexico border. She summarizes a list of the lessons learned for those interested in implementing similar programs among similar populations. In a review of health education activities at places of worship along the border, Kelly (Chapter 14) advocates recognizing the value of existing community structures for health promotion. He describes prior work and some current efforts to involve churches and religious organizations in health promotion. Challenging our notion of community as stable and specific to one location, Benavides-Vaello and Setzler (Chapter 15) document the range of health care concerns for those working with migrant and seasonal farmworker communities. Using data gathered from farmworkers and their families, the authors profile the individual and structural challenges to health care and prevention in this population.

The chapters in the volume are a selection of works that focus on a range of health issues pertinent to the U.S.-Mexico border region. As a selection, certain themes and emphases characterize the work represented. First, although submissions were solicited from researchers and practitioners working in Mexican institutions and agencies, the contributors in this volume are mainly affiliated with institutions in the United States. Consequently, the emphasis in the work represented is on research and practice as it is conducted and understood from the United States. We do not claim to represent the perspectives of those engaged in health research and practice on the Mexican side of the U.S.-Mexico border. Second, it would also be rather presumptuous of us to claim that we have addressed all facets of life that affect the health of border communities. Rather, we have selected a body of work that is diverse in terms of the range of topics and issues covered as well as the theoretical and methodological frameworks employed. There is also a diversity in the academic and professional backgrounds that inform the insights and perspectives represented. We believe that the combination of perspectives, methods, and disciplinary approaches is invaluable for understanding the complexity of health phenomena in the border region. Despite their diversity, there is also a consistent focus in the chapters in this volume on the uniqueness of the cultural, economic, and social elements that contribute to the health of the population living in the border region. Third, although the frame of reference is always the entire U.S.-Mexico border region, it is not surprising that many of our contributors have focused their attention on the El Paso/Ciudad Juárez metroplex. It is the largest urban region on the entire border, where many of the problems that prevail along the rest of the divide coalesce in one particular area. El Paso/Ciudad Juárez is also the busiest border crossing in the world and therefore serves as a valuable case study for health issues that arise at other international junctions throughout the world. Finally, the broad range of terms used to refer to ethnic groups, ethnic subgroups, and nationalities, such as *Hispanic, Mexican American, Mexican national,* and *Latino/Latina,* is represented in the chapters that follow. This breadth reflects the numerous referents used in studies cited in each chapter as well as the conventions of the respective authors. The U.S.-Mexico border has been described as a "caldron of poverty, pollution and neglect that threatens to spill its toxic brew nationwide" (Hearn, 1993, p. 13) and also as "the frontline where many of the issues that occupy this nation are being engaged" (Holley, 1994, p. 460). The problems in the border region are indeed overwhelming, and the consequences for those living in other regions of the United States and Mexico are great. However, much knowledge has been gleaned from the research and practice conducted by those who have taken on the challenges of border health. Some of that knowledge and the lessons learned are contained in the pages that follow. It is our hope that this compilation of research articles and practitioner reports will stimulate future interest in border health issues not only among researchers and practitioners but among policy makers and the population in general.

References

Bollini, P., & Siem, H. (1996). No real progress towards equity: Health of migrants and ethnic minorities on the eve of the year 2000. *Social Science and Medicine, 41,* 819-828.

Brown, S. A., & Hanis, C. L. (1995). A community-based, culturally sensitive education and group-support intervention for Mexican Americans with NIDDM: A pilot study of efficacy. *Diabetes Educator, 21,* 203-210.

Castillo, H. M. (1996). Cultural diversity: Implications for nursing. In S. Torres (Ed.), *Hispanic voices: Hispanic health educators speak out* (pp. 1-12). New York: NLN.

Dever, G. E. (1991). Migrant health status: Profile of a population with complex health problems. *Migrant Health Newsline: Monograph Series, 8*(2), 1-16.

El Paso Community Foundation. (1996). *The border/la frontera: The United States/Mexico international boundary.* El Paso, TX: Author.

Elshaw, E. B., Young, E. A., Saunders, M. J., McGurn, W. C., & Lopez, L. C. (1994). Utilizing a 24-hour dietary recall and culturally specific diabetes education in Mexican Americans with diabetes. *Diabetes Educator, 20,* 228-235.

Environmental Protection Agency. (1996). *U.S./Mexico Border XXI Program: Draft framework document* (EPA Pub. No. 160-D-96-001). Washington, DC: Author.

Guendelman, S., & Jasis, M. (1992). Giving birth across the border: The San Diego-Tijuana connection. *Social Science and Medicine, 34,* 419-425.

Ham-Chande, R., & Weeks, J. R. (1992). A demographic perspective of the U.S.-Mexico border. In J. R. Weeks & R. Ham-Chande (Eds.), *Demographic dynamics of the U.S.-Mexico border.* El Paso: Texas Western Press.

Hearn, W. (1993, September 20). Borderline risks. *American Medical News*, p. 13.

Hibbeln, J. A. (1996). Special populations: Hispanic migrant workers. In S. Torres (Ed.), *Hispanic voices: Hispanic health educators speak out* (pp. 162-192). New York: NLN.

Holley, J. (1994) Confronting la frontera: Who's watching the boom along the border? *Columbia Journalism Review, 33*(1), 46.

Stoddard, E. R. (1987). *Maquila: Assembly plants in northern Mexico.* El Paso: Texas Western Press.

Suárez y Toriello, E., & Chávez, O. E. (1996). *Profile of the United States-México border.* El Paso, TX: Federation of Private Associations for Community Development.

United States Mexico Border Health Association. (1994). *Sister communities health profiles.* El Paso, TX: Author.

University of Texas System. (1994). *Texas-Mexico border county demographics and health statistics: 1994.* Edinburg: University of Texas System, Texas-Mexico Border Health Coordination Office.

Part 1

Cultural Values and Health Promotion in the Border Region

To promote certain health practices or to advance the benefits of certain health information or advice, it is necessary to understand the values that prevail in the groups one is trying to reach. Understanding a community's values helps us to understand the motivation to learn new information and to behave in certain ways. Values also reflect the relative importance of competence and morality within certain groups. The social psychologist Milton Rokeach advanced the notion that people have instrumental and terminal values that guide their decisions about day-to-day activities and about long-term objectives, respectively. The extent to which one value predominates over another will influence one's attitude and related behavior. For example, if personal pleasure is more highly valued than family security, then one is likely to express attitudes and behaviors consistent with that priority.

The importance of cultural values to health behavior has long been a factor in the design of health campaigns by international agencies working in less developed countries. The acknowledgment of how cultural values influence target groups has been key to the success of health campaigns designed to influence immunization practices, water purification,

1

contraception, and safer sex. Many would argue that U.S. health agencies have been more sensitive to cultural values in the international arena than they have in the domestic context. The ethnocentric assumption that the health promotion strategies that have worked in European American populations will also work with other racial and ethnic groups has long been challenged by researchers and practitioners who work closely with Hispanic, African American, and Asian groups in the United States. This challenge has been based on an awareness of the importance of cultural values to health behavior. The HIV/AIDS crisis extended this awareness to the general population with more public discussions of how different groups think about and engage in sexual practices. Groups varied in their beliefs about high-risk practices, the importance of family, the influence of religion, and the sanctity of marriage. These beliefs, in turn, influenced their attitudes and behaviors regarding sex and other health practices.

The four articles in this section focus their attention on how cultural values influence the health practices of Hispanics in particular. The authors draw on a broad spectrum of evidence, gathered using different empirical methods and built on research literature from a variety of fields. They all explore how certain beliefs regarding the importance of family, the individual, friends, and language influence how Hispanics respond to health messages and their willingness to participate in health programs. The research findings are interpreted in the context of the U.S.-Mexico border environment, accounting for differences in class, language proficiency, and immigrant status where appropriate.

Chapter 1

∽∾

A MILE AWAY AND
A WORLD APART

The Impact of Interdependent and
Independent Views of the Self on
U.S.-Mexican Communications

SHEILA MURPHY

The way in which we think of ourselves in relation to others can dramatically shape the way we structure our communications, our relationships, and our lives. A growing body of research suggests that our view of ourselves—alternately referred to as our *self-construal, self-schema, self-concept,* or *self-orientation*—may not be universally shared but rather may be heavily dependent on cultural context. For example, Markus and Kitayama (1994) argued that although most cultures place some value on both individual autonomy and the good of the group, the relative emphasis placed on individualism and collectivism can vary dramatically across cultures. They noted that Western cultures such as the United States tend to extol the virtues of independence, personal achievement, and the development and maintenance of a separate and unique identity. Markus and Kitayama juxtaposed this Western worldview against that of Eastern cultures, where people tend to view themselves not as individuals but as fundamentally interconnected with others, rather like a single thread woven into an intricate fabric. Consequently, the focus in Eastern cultures is one

3

of the "self-in-relation-to-other people," in which the self is virtually defined by group membership and interpersonal relationships. Thus, according to Markus and Kitayama, Western cultures tend to emphasize the individual and being *independent* by asserting one's rights and showcasing one's unique talents and abilities (see also Shweder & Bourne, 1984), whereas Eastern cultures tend to stress *interdependence,* or maintaining group harmony and relationships (see also Bond, 1986; Hui, 1988; Miller, 1988).

These divergent views of self are more than passive cognitive representations. Rather, they play a pivotal role in motivating and regulating behavior (Markus & Wurf, 1987). The behaviors of an individual with a more independent worldview are guided by the individual's own thoughts, feelings, and actions. Individuals are expected to become self-reliant, ensuring that their own needs are met. The behaviors of an individual who has an interdependent self-construal, in contrast, are determined by a consideration of the thoughts, feelings, and actions of others with whom the individual has a social relationship. Thus, in interdependent cultures, group or family needs are typically placed above the needs of the individual (Triandis, Brislin, & Hui, 1988).

An independent or interdependent self-construal is often seen as the individual-level manifestation of an emphasis placed on individualism or collectivism at the national level (Gudykunst, Matsumoto, Ting-Toomey, Nishida, & Heyman, 1994). Yet as Markus and Kitayama (1994) were careful to point out, these orientations should be regarded as general tendencies that emerge when members of a particular culture are considered as a whole. Consequently, although a particular self-orientation may be predominant in a given culture, there will be considerable variation among individual members. Moreover, there may be dimensions other than independent-interdependent that also differentiate between cultures, such as the need for approval or the need for control (Salzman & Hunter, 1983). These issues notwithstanding, the premise of the present chapter is that, like the Eastern cultures described by Markus and Kitayama, Mexican culture may promote a more interdependent or collectivist self-orientation that may at times be at odds with the predominantly independent worldview of the United States.

What are the consequences of these divergent self-orientations for interpersonal communication generally and for health care communication more specifically? As Witte and Morrison (1995) pointed out,

> Meaning, or understanding, is often influenced by the communication context and the interpretive assumptions that each person holds. In the

health context, members of different cultures often bring different sets of interpretive assumptions to a communication interaction. For health professionals to help their patients or audiences, they must understand the interpretive frameworks within which their clients communicate. (p. 216)

A failure to recognize and be sensitive to alternate self-construals may result in rampant confusion, expectancy violation (Burgoon, 1995), and miscommunication. The remainder of this chapter attempts to show how Markus and Kitayama's (1991, 1994) theoretical framework regarding independent and interdependent self-construals may provide valuable insight into problems that commonly arise in health care communications along the U.S.-Mexico border. More specifically, the chapter will focus on two major sites of potential miscommunication—end-of-life decision making and sexual decision making—to illustrate how beliefs and behaviors that violate the normative expectations of an independent worldview might be better understood from an interdependent vantage point.

End-of-Life Decision Making

As discussed previously, the defining difference between an independent and an interdependent view of the self is the extent to which others are integrated into one's self-concept. Although others play a crucial role in any self-schema, individuals having an interdependent orientation see themselves as being defined primarily through their relationship with others (e.g., self as mother, coworker, or friend). One outgrowth of this emphasis on relationships is that individuals from interdependent cultures tend to be acutely aware of the feelings of those with whom they interact. From an early age, one learns not to burden others with one's problems. As a consequence, individuals from interdependent cultures tend to ignore or downplay illness as long as possible (Geissler, 1994). Such stoicism is evident in Mexican culture, particularly among Mexican males, for whom health is seen as an indicator of strength and manhood (Haffner, 1992). Mexicans, particularly those from rural areas, may turn to folk medicine first and to Western-style medicine only as a last resort (see Witte & Morrison, 1995, for a discussion of medical pluralism). As a result, diseases such as cancer or diabetes have often progressed much further among patients of Mexican descent by the time they first seek formal medical attention. In fact, it is not uncommon that by the time Mexican patients present themselves for treatment, they are close to death.

The issue of how terminal illness is handled is a prime example of the different worldviews that operate in U.S. and Mexican culture. Physicians in the United States strictly adhere to the principle of patient autonomy, which requires that the patient make informed decisions about his or her own medical care. In other words, patients should be fully informed about even fatal illnesses, be told the risks and benefits of proposed treatment options, and be allowed to make choices based on this information. Consequently, in the United States, it is standard practice for the doctor first to inform the patient of his or her diagnosis and prognosis, leaving it to the discretion of the patient whether to inform family members. Individuals from cultures having more interdependent orientations, such as Mexico, tend to prefer the exact opposite sequence of events—namely, first informing the family and leaving it to their discretion whether to inform the patient.

Thus, whereas those with independent orientations feel that the patient should be informed of a terminal diagnosis, individuals with more interdependent orientations feel that the patient should be protected from this news at all costs (Lock, 1983). This distinction was borne out in a study that my colleagues and I conducted (Blackhall, Murphy, Frank, Michel, & Azen, 1995). In the first year of this study, we conducted structured quantitative interviews with 800 individuals over the age of 65 living in the Los Angeles area—200 of Mexican descent, 200 of African descent, 200 of Korean descent, and 200 of European descent. These interviews were performed in the respondents' primary language. In the second year, ethnically matched anthropologists who specialize in each of these four ethnic groups performed in-depth ethnographic interviews with 10% of the original sample, providing context to the earlier quantitative data. These interviews covered a wide range of topics, from general attitudes toward Western medicine to more specific attitudes regarding end-of-life decision making. Of specific interest for present purposes are the differences between the Mexican[1] and European American respondents toward disclosure of a diagnosis and prognosis of a terminal illness and toward end-of-life decision making.

As shown in Table 1.1, individuals of Mexican descent were far less likely to agree that a patient should be told the diagnosis of cancer (48%) than individuals of European descent (87%). Moreover, less than half of our Mexican respondents felt that the doctor should reveal a terminal prognosis to the patient (48% compared to 69% for the European Americans). With regard to the question of whether to keep the patient alive on life support, Mexican respondents were more likely to nominate the family (45%) than the patient (41%) as the primary decision maker.[2] These results

TABLE 1.1 Degree of Patient Autonomy as a Function of Ethnicity

	European American	Mexican American	Korean American	African American
Physician should tell patient about metastatic cancer diagnosis[a]	87%[a]	48%[b]	35%[c]	89%[a]
Physician should tell patient about terminal prognosis[b]	69%[a]	48%[b]	35%[c]	63%[ab]
Who should make decision on life-prolonging technology:				
Patient	65%[a]	41%[bc]	28%[c]	60%[ab]
Family	20%[a]	45%[b]	57%[b]	24%[a]

NOTE: Percentages in the same row that do not share subscripts differ at $p < .05$.
a. "A doctor diagnoses a person as having cancer that has spread to several parts of their body. The doctor believes that the cancer cannot be cured. Should the doctor tell the patient that he or she has cancer?" (percentage answering yes).
b. "The doctor believes that the patient will probably die. Should the doctor tell the patient that he or she will probably die?" (percentage answering yes).
c. "The patient becomes very ill, and a decision must be made about whether to put the patient on life-prolonging machines. The machines will prolong the patient's life for a little while but will not cure the illness and may be uncomfortable. Who should make the decision about whether the patient is put on the machine?"

suggest that Mexican culture may promote a more family-centered model of medical decision making that runs counter to the prevailing U.S. model of patient autonomy.

One could argue that this pattern of findings is due, not to differing self-orientations, but rather to differences in social class. This was not the case. Great care was taken to recruit individuals in each of the four ethnic groups with roughly equivalent levels of education and income. Moreover, statistical analyses that hold income and education constant across the four ethnic groups reveal that ethnicity, not socioeconomic status, is the factor that underlies this pattern of results.

Indeed, some of our Mexican respondents thought it strange that the doctor would ask a patient to make this decision and suggested that perhaps this was a sign of incompetence. As Haffner (1992) noted, Mexicans typically "expect physicians to make the decisions for them and do not understand why they are asked to make choices. They are used to, and seem to prefer, deferring to experts" (p. 257). Our Mexican respondents also had a difficult time comprehending why a doctor would offer a seemingly futile treatment such as mechanical ventilation. Many resolved their dissonance by concluding that although the treatment was described in pessimistic terms, the doctor must actually believe that the mechanical ventilation could provide some benefit to the patient because he certainly would not waste such a valuable medical resource. This logic led some of our respondents to the interpretation that perhaps the doctor held out hope for recovery after all. It is easy to understand how such an interpretation could lead patients and their families to accept what is, in reality, futile treatment.

Along related lines, many respondents felt that they must not decline any treatment that a doctor suggests. This is consistent with Haffner's (1992) assertion that "Latinos[3] feel that they should agree with physicians out of respect, even when they really disagree or do not understand the issues involved" (p. 257). This politeness and respect norm can lead physicians to conclude erroneously that the patient and family are in agreement on a proposed course of action when in actuality they are strongly opposed (Klessig, 1992).

This overarching concern for the feelings of others is consistent with an interdependent construal of self. In Japan, for instance, there are strict cultural prohibitions against disturbing the *wa,* or the harmonious flow of social relations (Markus & Kitayama, 1991). A similar concept, *simpatia,* in Mexican culture "mandates politeness and respect and discourages assertiveness, direct negative responses, and criticism" (Lifshitz, 1990, p. 17). *Simpatia* involves respecting and empathizing with the feelings of others and remaining agreeable even under difficult circumstances (Church, 1987; Triandis, Marin, Lisansky, & Betancourt, 1984).

Simpatia is clearly evident in the reaction of Mexican family members to a patient. Someone who is ill is seen as incapable of making decisions (Muller & Desmond, 1992). Moreover, if the prognosis is grim, the patient must be shielded from the truth. The following excerpt from Haffner (1992), which describes a typical day in a Texas hospital, illustrates this point:

> When I arrive, the patient's family is distraught. They request a conference out of the patient's presence. The physician tells the family that the mother is dying and needs radical surgery, but he emphasizes that the surgery would prolong her life only a little. The physician wants to tell the patient and ask for her consent to the operation. The daughters are very upset and against saying anything to their mother. They beg me to explain that their mother has the right to have hopes, that she should not be told that she is going to die, and that a painful and difficult operation that may buy her

only a little more time is cruel. The result is an impasse that goes on for several days. The daughters vigilantly watch their mother, guarding her from the physicians, and hiding the truth from her. (p. 257)

Even in the face of terminal illness, the illusion of health is maintained by the family. Although at some level both the patient and the family realize that death is imminent, the family will assure the patient that he or she is "looking better" and "will be ready to return home soon." These practices, which are mandatory in Mexican culture, are in direct conflict with the Western medical establishment's ideal of patient autonomy and informed consent. This culture clash may be further exacerbated by the tendency of cultures that foster independent self-construals to favor very direct and linear forms of communication that "get straight to the point" and avoid "beating around the bush." Interdependent cultures, on the other hand, tend to favor a more indirect and subtle form of communication and perceive a direct recitation of the facts as cold and uncaring (Kim, 1995).

It is also noteworthy that the concept of "family" often varies as a function of self-orientation. In independent cultures such as the United States, the term *family* is commonly used in reference to one's nuclear family—namely, parents, siblings, and perhaps grandparents. Within interdependent cultures such as Mexico, however, the term has a much broader meaning. First, second, and possibly even third cousins may be included, as well as several friends of the family who are not connected by either blood or marriage. Consequently, the number of individuals who feel they have a right to be involved in the patient's health care decisions may vary dramatically by culture.

This is not to suggest that the more interdependent family-centered model of decision making is democratic. Rather, authority runs from oldest to youngest and from male to female, with the eldest male expected to receive diagnoses and make decisions regarding treatment for females and younger males (Haffner, 1992). Many physicians in the United States are taken aback to discover that a Mexican mother may not feel she has the authority to make decisions regarding medical treatment for herself or for her child (Geissler, 1994; Rasinski, 1993). Moreover, in Mexico, this patriarchal hierarchy is observed throughout the life span, with older adults continuing to make health care decisions for their adult children (Poma, 1987).

Such deference to one's elders and the past is common among societies with a predominantly interdependent orientation (Markus & Kitayama, 1991, 1994). Cultures that have a more independent worldview, in contrast, often have a more future orientation. It is no accident that the notion of advance care planning, which allows individuals to retain control over their fate even when unconscious, was conceived in the United States. Advance care directives for health care have been widely promoted as a way to improve end-of-life decision making. These documents allow a patient to state, in advance of incapacity, the types of medical treatments he or she would like to receive (a "living will"), to name a surrogate to make those decisions (a durable power of attorney for health care), or both. The principle of patient autonomy is so ingrained in the more independent U.S. culture that the benefits of such advance care planning seem obvious. Indeed, it has been argued that if individuals simply had sufficient information about and access to advance directives for health care, such as a living will or a durable power of attorney, they would complete them (Emanuel, Barry, Stoeckle, Ettleson, & Emanuel, 1991). To test the validity of this statement, my colleagues and I (Blackhall et al., 1995) asked the following question: If all individuals were equally educated with regard to advance directives, and if the requisite documents were readily available, would we see a uniformly high completion rate across all ethnic groups?

Our results, presented in Table 1.2, suggest that planning ahead may be a value associated with a more independent self-orientation (see also Lipson & Meleis, 1983). Although a complete lack of knowledge virtually precludes possessing either a living will or a durable power of attorney for health care, having knowledge ensures neither a positive attitude toward nor possession of an advance care directive. Our 200 Mexican respondents, despite a fairly high level of knowledge (47%), expressed a negative attitude toward written directives and had a fairly low rate of possession (10%). Those respondents who actually possessed a directive tended to have lived for a long time in the United States and were significantly more acculturated, as measured by Marin's Short Acculturation Scale (see Murphy et al., 1996, for more detail).

Compared to European Americans, Mexicans as a group had a negative attitude toward the concept of advance decision making. Two thirds of our Mexican American respondents endorsed items such as "Doctors should not discuss death and dying with their patients because it could be harmful to the patient" and "It is not necessary for people to write down their wishes about medical care because their family will know what to do when the time comes," compared to less than one third of their European American counterparts. These results further support the contention that Mexicans tend to place greater emphasis on family-centered, as opposed to patient-centered, decision-making styles (Blackhall et al., 1995).

TABLE 1.2 Knowledge and Possession of Advance Care Directives as a
Function of Ethnicity

	% With Knowledge of Either a Living Will or a Durable Power of Attorney for Health Care	% Who Possessed Either a Living Will or a Durable Power of Attorney for Health Care
Mexican Americans	47	10
European Americans	69	28
Korean Americans	13	0
African Americans	12	2

Even after the concept of advance care planning was explained and the requisite forms provided, respondents of Mexican descent were decidedly uninterested in completing an advance care directive. This outright rejection was probed further in subsequent ethnographic interviews. When asked why they felt negatively about advance care planning, the Mexican respondents frequently mentioned a sense that the future was in God's hands and that assuming that one could "plan" one's death was an affront to God—an affront for which he might seek retribution. This resonates with Klessig's (1992) assessment that for Mexicans, "Health is a gift from God, and ill health, including accidents, may be due to punishment from God or the saints. The suffering incurred is part of God's plan and should not be interfered with" (p. 321).

God and religion play a major role in Mexican health care beliefs and practices. When asked to state their preferences with regard to medical treatment, a common response among our Mexican respondents was "if God wants" ("si Diós quiere"). Physicians in the United States often mistakenly interpret this response as indicating that the patient does not want any medical intervention. This is not necessarily the case. As discussed previously, patients of Mexican descent may be uneasy when asked for input with regard to their medical treatment, feeling instead that God, or the doctor, should make the decision. Unfortunately, a strong belief in fate and God's omnipotence tends to be negatively correlated with perceptions of self-efficacy and control over one's life (Bandura, 1989). Witte and Morrison (1995) proposed that such a perceived lack of control may result in a fatalistic outlook and diminished health care with individuals espousing a "when it's my time to go, it's my time to go" (p. 239) attitude. This fatalistic attitude has dire implications for the ability of health care professionals or health campaigns to change behavior, for individuals who believe that they have no control over their future will not be motivated to adhere to a treatment regimen or to alter their current activities and lifestyle.

Sexual Decision Making

This perceived lack of control over one's fate is evident in the response, or lack thereof, among individuals of Mexican descent to the AIDS epidemic. The rate of human immunodeficiency virus (HIV) infection for individuals of Mexican descent is among the fastest growing in the nation (Centers for Disease Control and Prevention [CDC], 1995). Although they constitute only 8% of the population, this group represents 16% of reported AIDS cases nationally (CDC, 1995). In other words, among known HIV cases, individuals of Mexican descent are dramatically overrepresented with respect to their prevalence in the general population.

A variety of cultural and economic factors have been posited to explain the elevated rate of HIV among both Mexicans and Mexican Americans (Hernandez & Smith, 1990; Maldonado, 1990; Marin, 1990). Marin (1990) pointed to the double standard that exists in Mexican culture with regard to sexuality. Mexican men are often encouraged to have sex at an early age and to have multiple sexual partners, whereas women are differentiated into those who are"good" (e.g., faithful to a single partner) and those who are "bad" (e.g., sexually available outside marriage or stable relationships). Marin asserted that this double standard may serve to constrain the sexual activity of most women while increasing the sexual activity of men. As Klein and Wolf (1985) pointed out, this "good-bad" categorization of women may result in men's perceiving that wives, or women who may become their wives (novias), are not prime sexual targets and instead turning to other available partners to demonstrate "virility" (Carrier, 1985), including both male[4] (Klein & Wolf, 1985) and female sex workers, who are at particularly high risk for carrying the HIV virus (Peterson & Marin, 1988).

Consequently, for women of Mexican descent, a major source of HIV transmission is apt to involve the risky behavior of their male partner. An obvious solution to this problem is to encourage women to persuade their partners to use condoms. Unfortunately, condom use remains particularly low among this population (DiClemente, 1991; Moore, Harrison, & Doll,

1994; Weinstock, Lindan, Bolan, Kegeles, & Hearst, 1993). In one study for the CDC, over 40% of Latinas reported that they would have sex without a condom with a partner who was HIV positive, compared to only 15% of European American women (Harrison et al., 1991, cited in Moore et al., 1994). Unfortunately, this low incidence of condom use is reflected in the relatively high seroprevalence rate among Mexican American women. Over 20% of the women diagnosed with AIDS are Latina (CDC, 1995), although Latinas represent only 6% of the U.S. population (U.S. Bureau of the Census, 1990).[5]

In Latin American cultures generally, value systems may make negotiating safer sex problematic. First, discussions of sexual matters between men and women are often considered taboo, even between husbands and wives (Marin, 1990). Men of Mexican descent find it particularly difficult to talk about sexual matters (Marin, 1990). It has been suggested that Latinos may be reluctant to disclose their HIV status to their partners because they fear rejection and loss of emotional support (Des Jarlais, Chamberland, Yancovitz, Weinberg, & Friedman, 1994). This is, of course, consistent with an interdependent orientation, in which relationships are valued above all else. This silence, however, has deadly consequences. As Peterson and Marin (1988) pointed out, because Latinos do not disclose their sexual histories readily, the sexual partners of HIV-positive men may incorrectly assume that they are not at risk.

As might be expected from an interdependent orientation, Mexican women are extremely sensitive to the feelings, needs, and desires of their partners. For example, Weinstock et al. (1993) found that Mexican women are especially unlikely to use condoms when their partners respond negatively to their use. Marin (1990) suggested that the direct confrontation that might be necessary in insisting that one's partner use a condom is at odds with the cultural value of *simpatia,* which stresses the importance of smooth interpersonal relations (Triandis et al., 1984). Direct challenges to male partners regarding condom use may also be perceived as threatening *machismo* (Marin, 1990) and may result in rejection, abuse, or even accusations of infidelity.[6] Furthermore, as Maldonado (1990) argued, Latinas who are economically and emotionally dependent on their partners are unlikely to insist on condom use if their male partners resist.

Cultural beliefs that women should not be knowledgeable about sex may likewise reduce the motivation to seek out information about AIDS. In fact, knowledge regarding AIDS, as well as beliefs that using condoms can be an effective preventative measure against HIV, was significantly lower for Spanish-speaking compared to English-speaking women in family planning clinics, even though information was provided in both Spanish and English (Rapkin & Erikson, 1990). But this lack of AIDS-related information is not limited to women. DiClemente, Boyer, and Morales (1988), in a study of high-risk adolescent males in San Francisco, found that white students were more knowledgeable about AIDS than were black students, who in turn were more knowledgeable than Latino students. Latinos also scored significantly lower in terms of AIDS knowledge on the 1988 National Survey of Adolescent Males (Sonenstein, Pleck, & Leighton, 1989).

What accounts for these relatively low levels of AIDS knowledge among Latinos? Similar trends have been found with regard to knowledge about sex and contraceptive use, suggesting that it is not AIDS per se that is a taboo topic but issues of sexuality more generally (Padilla & O'Grady, 1987). One especially relevant study examined contraceptive use and pregnancy among 300 women living on each side of the U.S.-Mexico border in the twin cities of El Paso and Juárez (Russell, Williams, Farr, Schwab, & Plattsmier, 1993). Whereas 94% of the women in El Paso, Texas, reported that they had heard about condoms, this was true for only 75% of the women in Juárez. In terms of actual use, the gap was even more dramatic, with almost twice as many of the women in El Paso reporting having used a condom (19.3% vs. 10.2% in Juárez). Furthermore, the most commonly used method of birth control in Juárez was the rhythm method (26.4%), whereas the most common method in El Paso was the pill (12%). Interestingly, women in Juárez also tended to hold the opinion that birth control methods are bad for one's health and that they are generally unreliable. Finally, whereas women in El Paso reported using birth control to avoid pregnancy, those in Juárez tended to frame birth control as a way to optimize the timing of children to ensure their health. Notice that these divergent explanations are consistent with the proposed independent (i.e., avoid getting pregnant) and interdependent (i.e., ensure health of child) views of self.

In sum, a fatalistic attitude about the future, a sense that illness may be a retribution for one's sins, religious prohibitions against condoms, a heavy emphasis on procreation, a reluctance to discuss sex or sexual history, and other associated behaviors and beliefs appear to result in a relatively low level of knowledge and a relatively high incidence of HIV. This constellation of cultural beliefs and practices presents quite a challenge for health care communication. The following section examines how being sensitive to divergent construals of self might make attitude change campaigns more efficacious.

Implications for Health Care Campaigns

Although much research has been directed at identifying factors that motivate people to protect themselves against health risk, the bulk of this research has targeted white middle-class Americans (Witte & Morrison, 1995). Not surprisingly, therefore, the vast majority of health care campaigns reflect an independent orientation. Typically, these health care campaigns attempt to coax the individual to engage in positive behaviors by appealing to his or her self-interest. This assertion was supported by a content analysis conducted by my colleague, Lynn Miller, and myself in conjunction with the CDC. We content-analyzed 101 television public service announcements, 45 radio spots, and 19 clinic brochures available in the greater Los Angeles area dealing with AIDS. Our analysis determined that the vast majority of these messages were independent in orientation in that they attempted to induce attitude and behavior change by appealing to the individual to act in his or her own best interest by "looking out for Number 1." In fact, the primary theme in over 75% of messages in each of these three media was "protect yourself" (see Miller, Murphy, & Clark, 1996, for details).

Although "protect yourself" may be an effective message in cultures that stress independence and self-efficacy, it may be substantially less effective in cultures that promote a more interdependent worldview. To individuals of Mexican descent who place heavy emphasis on relationships and family, messages that appeal to self-interest, such as "protect yourself," seem strange at best. Because these messages are at odds with their predominant cultural beliefs and values, it is unlikely that members of more interdependent cultures would possess either the motivation or the ability to integrate them into their everyday lives.

Messages that hope to motivate by appealing to self-interest may be particularly problematic for women. As alluded to previously, there is empirical evidence to suggest that the degree to which one ascribes to an independent orientation also varies *within* cultures (Markus & Kitayama, 1994). One fairly consistent finding is that women, regardless of cultural orientation, tend to be more likely to define themselves in terms of relationships (e.g., mother, sister) than men (Gilligan 1982; Jordan, Kaplan, Miller, Stivey, & Surrey, 1991) and to be especially concerned with maintaining relationships. That females in general would tend to be more interdependent in orientation makes intuitive sense in that traditional sex roles seem to parallel the independent-interdependent self orientations.

Whereas males tend to evaluate themselves on independent dimensions such as competition, individual achievement, and dominance, the female sense of self tends to be measured by the more interdependent traits of caring, cooperation, and empathy (Gilligan, 1982, 1987). Research also suggests that members of marginalized groups (e.g., nondominant ethnic groups, the poor, the unschooled, the elderly) share a more interdependent or group orientation (Markus & Kitayama, 1994). Thus, although independent-interdependent orientations may provide a useful tool to understand differences at the cultural level, we must bear in mind that there is substantial within-group variation and that some subgroups of the population may constitute cultures in their own right (Maltz & Borker, 1982).

Taken together, these findings should lead us to question the utility of health care messages that are individualistic in orientation for women generally and for Mexican women in particular. Lynn Miller and I are currently collecting data to address this issue. To identify the goals that these women see as most relevant to them, we asked Mexican and Mexican American women living in the Los Angeles area to list three things that they considered the most important in the world, three things that they hoped would happen in their life, and three things that they feared would happen. Whereas our content analysis revealed that the majority of the AIDS-related messages on TV, on the radio, and in clinic brochures in this area had a heavy independent emphasis ("protect yourself"), our respondents appeared to be far more likely to mention collectivist or interdependent themes such as protecting loved ones.

Although these data are preliminary, they suggest that in the Mexican community, the values of cooperation, community, and family responsibility might be more efficacious motivators in health appeals (see also Marin & Marin, 1991; Mays & Cochran, 1988). Effective messages must also enable women to circumnavigate intrapersonal, interpersonal, and cultural obstacles. For example, *machismo* might be harnessed in AIDS prevention campaigns by stressing the role of men as providers and protectors of the family (Marin, 1990). Also, Marin (1990) and Lifshitz (1990) suggested that rather than directly confronting religious beliefs regarding condom use, health care appeals tap into a major motivational source for Latinas— namely, staying healthy to continue to care adequately for their children. "Anything that jeopardizes her life also jeopardizes the well-being of her offspring. That awareness may provide the leverage that could persuade her to reconsider her feelings against condom use" (Lifshitz, 1990, p. 17). Perhaps a more effective message for this audience might involve more interdependent goals: for example, "Protect your loved ones" or "Who would take care of your family if something happened to you?"

According to Markus and her colleagues (Markus & Kitayama, 1991, 1994; Markus & Wurf, 1987), motivating individuals to action is an important function of the self-concept. Unfortunately, there is little systematic work examining how individuals with different self-orientations process health care messages and incorporate recommendations into their everyday lives. However, if we extrapolate from extant research, we might predict that individuals with an independent view of self would be motivated to act in ways that allowed them to express their self-defining inner attributes, such as being creative, autonomous, or unique. In contrast, individuals with a more interdependent orientation might be more likely to act on messages that allowed them to express feelings of relatedness or connectedness to others.

Conclusion

The premise of this chapter was that the United States, with its emphasis on freedom, equality, and individual rights, tends to foster an independent construal of self, whereas Mexico, with its reverence for family and its notion of *simpatia,* may promote a more interdependent construal of self. It was further argued that these divergent perspectives may result in intercultural confusion and miscommunication. A review of the relevant research seems to support these contentions.

It is important to bear in mind, however, that although independent versus interdependent self-orientations may provide a useful heuristic in understanding differences between cultures, it is a relatively gross categorization and, as such, is unlikely to characterize adequately every individual in every situation. Obviously, there are individuals within a given culture for whom these general self-construals do not apply. Nor should we expect an individual always to act in accordance with his or her primary self-construal.

Moreover, for the sake of simplicity, the present chapter focused primarily on a conception of self as put forward by Markus and Kitayama (1991), in which a culture tends to emphasize and promote either a predominantly independent value system or a predominantly interdependent value system. The relative weight assigned these value systems at the cultural level tends to be reflected in the self-orientations of its members. This is not to say that individuals cannot possess both value systems. Indeed, Triandis (1989) argued that these two aspects of self can coexist and emerge in different situations. For example, he suggested that a view of ourselves as independent may be more likely to emerge and guide our actions when we are alone, whereas our interdependent view of self may be more accessible when in-groups are salient (Triandis, McCusker, & Hui, 1990).[7] The idea of more than one self-construal coexisting is not necessarily inconsistent with Markus and Kitayama's theoretical framework. Indeed, they explicitly stated that cultures and individuals possess both value systems to some extent and that which of the two self-construals— independent or interdependent—is more chronically accessible to the individual and therefore more likely to influence behavior tends to vary by culture.

The issue of whether the independent and interdependent aspects of self are orthogonal may have interesting implications with regard to the issue of acculturation. Shibutani and Kwan (1965) defined acculturation as the process of learning and acquiring some, but not all, aspects of a host culture. This raises an intriguing issue: Does acquiring elements of a new host culture necessitate "deculturation" from one's former culture? There is scant research with which to address this question. In one relevant study, Cross and Markus (1991) examined the self-construals of East Asian exchange students. Their results indicate that living in the United States resulted in an increase in the value that these students placed on independence but did not decrease the value they placed on interdependence. This seems to imply that independent and interdependent self-construals may be orthogonal and consequently can coexist. On the other hand, Russell et al.'s (1993) previously cited study of contraceptive use and pregnancy among young women along the U.S.-Mexico border suggests that although the physical distance between El Paso and Juárez is less than a mile, the psychological distance may be much further.

Many questions remain unanswered. For example, if an individual develops two distinct self-orientations, one that predominates in his or her native land and one that is stressed in the adopted land, which is likely to be more influential in terms of health care decisions? Barker (1992) argued that "no matter how acculturated a person appears, at times of great stress, such as illness or death, early-learned ideas resurface and structure responses" (p. 251). Although this has intuitive merit, there are no data either to support or to refute this assertion.

Finally, must acculturation involve a physical move to another country, or can it occur through constant mass media exposure to the values, beliefs, and behaviors of another culture? The mass media of host countries have been shown to facilitate the adaptation and acculturation of immigrants (Subervi-Velez, 1986). Moreover, Kang, Kapoor, and Wolfe (1996) found that among Indian viewers, support of individualistic values increased as a function of the amount of time they spent viewing U.S. television programs. It may follow, therefore, that chronic exposure to a diet of mass media programming from a predominantly independent culture may substantially influence the self-orientation of interdependent viewers and vice versa.

Perhaps independent and interdependent views of self will provide a useful framework to address these and other questions. Clearly, further work is needed. It is important to keep in mind, however, that the purpose of distinguishing between independent and interdependent views of self is not to draw attention to differences and perpetuate cultural stereotypes. Rather, the goal is to sensitize readers and health care professionals to the cultural contexts and differing worldviews that individuals carry with them when they cross the border.

Notes

1. We refer to our respondents as "Mexican Americans," although the group consisted almost exclusively of Mexican nationals who had lived in the United States for various periods of time.

2. It is interesting to note the similarity between the responses of the Mexican and the Korean groups, both of whom appear to subscribe to a family-centered model of medical decision making. This similarity supports our contention that Mexican culture, like many Asian cultures, promotes an interdependent construal of self.

3. I am somewhat uncomfortable with the use of the terms *Latino* and *Latina* because they seem to clump individuals from many countries together, ignoring what may be significant cultural differences between Latin American subgroups (e.g., Cubans, Puerto Ricans, Mexicans). Though I prefer grouping individuals in clusters no larger than country of origin, Marin (1990) and others have argued that although there may be a number of important differences between Latin American countries, there is also significant overlap, suggesting that the single term may be acceptable. Although I agree that many cultures in Latin America share an interdependent orientation, I will use the more specific terms *Mexican* and *Mexican American* unless referring to research that employs the term *Latino*.

4. Interestingly, in Mexican culture it is not taboo for a man to engage in sex with a male prostitute. As long as the client is in the insertive role, this is not seen as a reflection on his own sexual orientation.

5. Unfortunately, male-to-female transmission appears to be an especially effective conduit, and women—83% of whom have contracted HIV through heterosexual sex—are currently one of the fastest growing segments of the AIDS epidemic (CDC, 1995). By the year 2000, it is expected that the number of women infected will surpass the number of men.

6. With regard to tolerance for infidelity, there is also a double standard. A married woman's engaging in sex with a man other than her husband is strictly forbidden and harshly punished. When a man cheats on his wife, however, it is often ignored or tolerated as something that will

pass without undermining the wife's position. This is illustrated by the saying "There are many chapels [other women], but the cathedral [the wife] should not be jealous of the chapels."

7. Along similar lines, Argyle (1991) noted that a number of cross-cultural studies suggest that individualism and collectivism are not opposites but rather separate orthogonal factors. This framework suggests four possible types of cultures: one type in which both values are high, one type in which both values are low, and two types in which one value is high and the other low.

References

Argyle, M. (1991). *Cooperation: The nature of sociability.* London: Routledge.

Bandura, A. (1989). Perceived self-efficacy in the exercise of control over AIDS infection. In V. M. Mays, G. W. Albee, & S. F. Schneider (Eds.), *Primary prevention of AIDS: Psychological approaches* (pp. 128-141). Newbury Park, CA: Sage.

Barker, J. C. (1992). Cultural diversity: Changing the context of medical practice. *Western Journal of Medicine, 157,* 248-254.

Blackhall, L. J., Murphy, S. T., Frank, G., Michel, V., & Azen, S. (1995). Ethnicity and attitudes toward patient autonomy. *Journal of the American Medical Association, 247,* 820-825.

Bond, M. H. (1986). *The psychology of the Chinese people.* New York: Oxford University Press.

Burgoon, J. K. (1995). Cross-cultural and intercultural applications of expectancy violations theory. *International and Intercultural Communication Annual, 19,* 194-214.

Carrier, J. M. (1985). Mexican male bisexuality. In F. Klein & T. J. Wolf (Eds.), *Bisexualities: Theory and research* (pp. 75-85). New York: Hawthorn.

Centers for Disease Control and Prevention. (1995). *Division of HIV/AIDS Prevention annual report.* Atlanta: Author.

Church, A. T. (1987). Personality research in a non-Western culture: The Philippines. *Psychological Bulletin, 102,* 272-292.

Cross, S. E., & Markus, H. R. (1991). *Cultural adaptation and the self: Self-construal, coping and stress.* Paper presented at the annual meeting of the American Psychological Association, San Francisco.

Des Jarlais, D. C., Chamberland, M. E., Yancovitz, S. R., Weinberg, P., & Friedman, S. R. (1994). Heterosexual partners: A large risk group for AIDS. *Lancet, 2,* 1346-1347.

DiClemente, R. J. (1991). Predictors of HIV-preventive behavior in a high-risk adolescent population: The influence of perceived peer norms and sexual communication on incarcerated adolescents' consistent use of condoms. *Journal of Adolescent Health, 12,* 385-390.

DiClemente, R. J., Boyer, C. B., & Morales, E. (1988). Minorities and AIDS: A survey of knowledge, attitudes and beliefs about AIDS in San Francisco. *American Journal of Public Health, 76,* 1443-1445.

Emanuel, L. L., Barry, M. J., Stoeckle, J. D., Ettleson, L. M., & Emanuel, E. J. (1991). Advance directives for medical care: A case for greater use. *New England Journal of Medicine, 324,* 889-895.

Geissler, E. M. (1994). *Pocket guide to cultural assessment.* St. Louis, MO: C. V. Mosby.

Gilligan, C. (1982). *In a different voice: Psychological theory and women's development.* Cambridge, MA: Harvard University Press.

Gilligan, C. (1987). Moral orientation and moral development. In E. F. Kittay & D. T. Meyers (Eds.), *Women and moral theory* (pp. 19-33). Ottawa, NJ: Rowman & Littlefield.

Gudykunst, W. B. (1995). Anxiety/uncertainty management theory: Current status. *International and Intercultural Communication Annual, 19,* 8-58.

Gudykunst, W. B., Matsumoto, Y., Ting-Toomey, S., Nishida, T., & Heyman, S. (1994). *Measuring self-construals across cultures.* Paper presented at the International Communication Association Convention, Sydney, Australia.

Gudykunst, W. B. (1993). Toward a theory of effective interpersonal and intergroup communication: An anxiety/uncertainty management (AUM) perspective. In R. L. Wiseman & J. Koester (Eds.), *Intercultural communication competence* (pp. 19-39). Newbury Park, CA: Sage.

Gudykunst, W. B., Gao, G., Schmidt, K. L., Nishida, Y., Bond, M. H., Kwok, L., Wang, G., & Barraclough, R. A. (1992). The influence of individualism-collectivism, self-monitoring, and predicted outcome value on communication in ingroup outgroup relationships. *Journal of Cross-Cultural Psychology, 23,* 196-213.

Haffner, L. (1992). Translation is not enough: Interpreting in a medical setting. *Western Journal of Medicine, 157,* 255-259.

Hernandez, J. T., & Smith, F. J. (1990). Racial targeting of AIDS programs considered. *Journal of the National Medical Association, 83,* 17-21.

Hui, C. H. (1988). Measurement of individualism-collectivism. *Journal of Research on Personality, 22,* 17-36.

Jemmott, J. B., & Jones, J. M. (1993). Social psychology and AIDS among ethnic minority individuals: Risk behaviors and strategies for changing them. In J. Pryor & G. Reeder (Eds.), *The social psychology of HIV infection.* Hillsdale, NJ: Lawrence Erlbaum.

Jordan, J. V., Kaplan, A. G., Miller, J. B., Stivey, I. P., & Surrey, J. L. (Eds.). (1991). *Women's growth in connection.* New York: Guilford.

Kang, J., Kapoor, S. B., & Wolfe, A. (1996). The impact of television viewing on the value orientations of Indian students: An individualist-collectivist approach. *Howard Journal of Communication.*

Kim, M. S. (1995). Toward a theory of conversational constraints: Focusing on individual-level dimension of culture. *International and Intercultural Communication Annual, 19,* 148-169.

Kim, Y. K. (1995). Cross-cultural adaptation: An integrative theory. *International and Intercultural Communication Annual, 19,* 170-193.

Klein, F., & Wolf, T. J. (Eds.). (1985). *Bisexualities: Theory and research.* New York: Hawthorn.

Klessig, J. (1992). The effects of values and culture on life support decisions. *Western Journal of Medicine, 157,* 316-322.

Lifshitz, A. (1990, December). Critical cultural barriers that bar meeting the needs of Latinas. *SIECUS Report,* pp. 16-17.

Lipson, J. G., & Meleis, A. I. (1983). Issues in health care of Middle Eastern patients. *Western Journal of Medicine, 139,* 271-275.

Lock, M. (1983). Japanese responses to social change: Making the strange familiar. *Western Journal of Medicine, 139,* 25-30.

Maldonado, M. (1990, December). Latinas and HIV/AIDS: Implications for the 90s. *SIECUS Report,* pp. 11-15.

Maltz, D. N., & Borker, R. A. (1982). A cultural approach to male-female miscommunication. In J. J. Gumperz (Ed.), *Language and social identity* (pp. 196-216). New York: Cambridge University Press.

Marin, B. V. (1990). Hispanic culture: Implications for AIDS prevention. In J. Boswell, R. Hexter, & J. Reinisch (Eds.), *Sexuality and disease: Metaphors, perception and behavior in the AIDS era.* New York: Oxford University Press.

Marin, G., & Marin, B. V. (1991). *Research with Hispanic populations.* Newbury Park, CA: Sage.

Markus, H. R., & Kitayama, S. (1991). Culture and the self: Implications for cognition, emotion and motivation. *Psychological Review, 98,* 224-247.

Markus, H. R., & Kitayama, S. (1994). A collective fear of the collective: Implications of selves and theories of selves. *Personality and Social Psychology Bulletin, 20,* 568-579.

Markus, H. R., & Wurf, E. (1987). The dynamic self concept: A social psychological perspective. *Annual Review of Psychology, 38,* 299-337.

Mays, V. M., & Cochran, S. D. (1988). Issues in the perception of AIDS risk and risk reduction activities by black and Hispanic/Latina women. *American Psychologist, 43,* 949-957.

Miller, J. G. (1988). Bridging the content-structure dichotomy: Culture and the self. In M. M. Bond (Ed.), *The cross-cultural challenge to social psychology* (pp. 266-281). Newbury Park, CA: Sage.

Miller, L. C., Bettencourt, B. A., DeBro, S. C., & Hoffmann, V. (1993). Negotiating safer sex: An interpersonal process. In J. Pryor & G. Reeder (Eds.), *The social psychology of HIV infection.* Hillsdale, NJ: Lawrence Erlbaum.

Miller, L. C., Murphy, S. T., & Clark, L. (1996). *Selling safer sex: Do AIDS messages fit the everyday goals of high risk women?* Paper presented at the 11th International AIDS Conference, Vancouver, Canada.

Moore, J. S., Harrison, J. S., & Doll, L. S. (1994). Interventions for sexually active heterosexual women in the United States. In R. J. DiClemente & J. L. Peterson (Eds.), *Preventing AIDS: Theories and methods of behavioral interventions.* New York: Plenum.

Muller, J. H., & Desmond, B. (1992). Ethical dilemmas in a cross-cultural context: A Chinese example. *Western Journal of Medicine, 157,* 323-327.

Murphy, S. T., Palmer, J., Azen, S., Frank, G., Michel, V., & Blackhall, L. (1996). Ethnicity and advance care directives. *Journal of Law, Medicine and Ethics, 24,* 108-117.

Padilla, E. R., & O'Grady, K. E. (1987). Sexuality among Mexican Americans: A case of sexual stereotyping. *Journal of Personality and Social Psychology, 52,* 5-10.

Peterson, J. L., & Marin, G. (1988). Issues in the prevention of AIDS among black and Hispanic men. *American Psychologist, 43,* 871-877.

Poma, P. A. (1987). Pregnancy in Hispanic women. *Journal of the National Medical Association, 79,* 929-935.

Rapkin, A. J., & Erikson, P. I. (1990). Differences in knowledge of and risk factors for AIDS between Hispanic and non-Hispanic women attending an urban family planning clinic. *AIDS, 4,* 889-899.

Rasinski, D. (1993). Cross-cultural concerns and communication in health care. In B. C. Thornton & G. L. Kreps (Eds.), *Perspectives on health communication* (pp. 165-177). Prospect Heights, IL: Waveland.

Russell, A. Y., Williams, M. S., Farr, P. A., Schwab, J. A., & Plattsmier, S. (1993). Patterns of contraceptive use and pregnancy among young Hispanic women on the Texas-Mexico border. *Journal of Adolescent Health, 14,* 373-379.

Salzman, K., & Hunter, J. E. (1983). *The voicer/nonvoicer distinction: A dimension in the experience of conscious thought.* Unpublished manuscript.

Shibutani, T., & Kwan, K. (1965). *Ethnic stratification: A comparative approach.* New York: Macmillan.

Shweder, R. A., & Bourne, E. J. (1984). Does the concept of the person vary cross-culturally? In R. A. Shweder & R. A. LeVine (Eds.), *Culture theory: Essays on mind, self, and emotion* (pp. 158-199). New York: Cambridge University Press.

Sonenstein, F. L., Pleck, J. H., & Leighton, C. K. (1989). Sexual activity, condom use and AIDS awareness among adolescent males. *Family Planning Perspectives, 21,* 152-158.

Subervi-Velez, F. (1986). The mass media and ethnic assimilation and pluralism. *Communication Research, 13*(1), 71-76.

Triandis, T. (1989). The self and social behavior in differing cultural contexts. *Psychological Review, 96,* 506-520.

Triandis, T., Brislin, R., & Hui, C. H. (1988). Cross-cultural training across the individualism-collectivism divide. *International Journal of Intercultural Relations, 12,* 269-289.

Triandis, T., Marin, G., Lisansky, J., & Betancourt, H. (1984). Simpatico as a cultural script of Hispanics. *Journal of Personality and Social Psychology, 47,* 1365-1375.

U.S. Bureau of the Census. (1990). *Vital statistics.* Washington, DC: Government Printing Office.

Weinstock, H. S., Lindan, C., Bolan, G., Kegeles, S. M., & Hearst, N. (1993). Factors associated with condom use in a high-risk heterosexual population. *Sexually Transmitted Diseases, 20,* 14-20.

Witte, K., & Morrison, K. (1995). Intercultural and cross-cultural health communication: Understanding people and motivating healthy behaviors. *International and Intercultural Communication Annual, 19,* 216-246.

Chapter 2

⤬

INCREASING THE CONSENT RATE FOR ORGAN DONATION IN THE HISPANIC POPULATION

IRMA HINOJOSA

At present, more than 30,000 people are on a national waiting list for an organ transplant, and seven people die each day for lack of a suitable organ.

Evanisko, quoted in press release from the
Partnership for Organ Donation, Inc. ("Landmark
Survey Finds Organ Shortage Persists," 1993)

Despite the severe shortage of donated organs, 9 out of 10 Americans believe that organ donation allows something positive to come out of death (Gallup Organization, 1993). Support for organ donation is significantly lower among Hispanics than for non-Hispanic whites. The Southwest Organ Bank, Inc. was founded in 1974 to respond to the challenge of organ donation in the Southwest region of the United States. It is the first independent organ procurement organization in Texas. Headquartered in Dallas, Southwest Organ Bank has regional offices in six other Texas cities, with a service population of approximately 7 million. Organ transplant programs in Southwest Organ Bank's service areas include heart, heart and lung, kidney, liver, small bowel, and pancreas. This chapter documents the experiences of a regional coordinator in one Southwest Organ Bank facility in a Texas border town. I focus specifically on the cultural challenges to organ donation among the Hispanic population, where organ donation has traditionally been very low (Callender, Bey, Miles, & Yeager, 1995; Renee, Viera, Daniels, & Santos, 1994).

In 1993, the Partnership for Organ Donation and the Harvard School of Public Health commissioned a national survey of public attitudes toward organ donation. Although 72% of non-Hispanic whites said they would be very or somewhat likely to donate their organs on death, that figure dropped to 57% for Hispanics. The findings also highlighted a range of concerns about both donation and transplantation among respondents. Hispanics are more concerned than non-Hispanic whites about the disfigurement of the body after organ donation and about the need to be buried with all of the body's parts intact. Whereas 37% of non-Hispanic whites considered transplantation to be an experimental medical procedure, this figure rose to 46% among Hispanics. The incorrect belief that a brain-dead person—a potential organ donor—can recover is held by 19% of non-Hispanic whites and 29% of Hispanics. Gortmaker (quoted in press release from the Partnership for Organ Donation, Inc., "Minorities Less Supportive of Organ Donation Than Whites," March 30, 1993) suggested that the donor shortage cannot be solved without the participation of minorities and that this cannot be achieved without identifying and resolving the issues unique to minority communities.

Nationwide, Hispanics account for only 9% of the population. The census figures indicate that those numbers are rapidly increasing. In El Paso, Hispanics account for 69% of the 600,000 population of the city (U.S. Bureau of the Census, 1990). In the United States, only the Rio Grande valley area has a higher percentage of Hispanics. These numbers are due to the historical relationship and proximity of these areas to the border with Mexico. El Paso has strong ties with its sister city, Ciudad Juárez. Ciudad Juárez is twice the size of El Paso, and residents of both cities travel across the border daily. The residents of Juárez come to El Paso to shop, work, and obtain quality health care. The county hospital in El Paso serves as the only trauma center in a 250-mile radius and is sometimes the only source of health care for the over 1 million Mexican nationals living on the other side of the border. Although Hispanics represent the majority of the population in this community, in 1991 they accounted for 50% of the referrals made to Southwest Organ Bank and only 25% of the total donors recovered. This retrospective study documents the change in the consent rate among Hispanic families from 1991 to 1993.

I joined Southwest Organ Bank's El Paso staff in 1992. My background is in public relations and marketing. I have no formal training in the medical field. I am bilingual and have lived in El Paso most of my life. I am very familiar with the El Paso community. Many of the issues in El Paso are similar to those faced by coordinators approaching families across the country, especially families of a lower socioeconomic status. In 1989, the national average income for a Mexican American family was $29,564. In El Paso, the 1990 census showed the median family income to be approximately $24,000, which includes both Hispanics and non-Hispanics. Among Hispanics alone, the median income drops to $14,000. These families share a complex set of cultural characteristics that often inhibit their involvement in organ donation. Below, I identify these cultural characteristics and the strategies I have employed to address them.

Distrust of the Medical System

Many Hispanics of lower socioeconomic status feel uncomfortable with medical professionals and staff. Hospitals in El Paso, as in many other border cities, see Mexican patients in their emergency rooms. Often, this is the first encounter with the medical system for these Mexican families, and they are easily intimidated by physicians and other authority figures. These patients and their families may or may not be in the United States legally. Therefore, to protect themselves or family members not holding a current legal alien card, they will be reluctant to talk to physicians or other hospital staff. They may not give real names or addresses, and they often use fictitious social security numbers. It is helpful, therefore, to dissociate oneself from the hospital and its staff.

Strategy

I introduce myself to families as a representative of the Organ Bank—not a nurse or a medical person, but someone who is there to help them understand the unique situation that they are in. I emphasize that I am not concerned with their legal status and that I do not have any authority in that area. Thus, the distrust that many of these families have for the medical or legal system is not associated with me or the issues that I need to discuss with them. Although, in reality, the Organ Bank works very closely with the hospitals it serves, this strategy of separating the hospital staff from the Organ Bank staff is important. It is imperative that the hospital staff maintain their role as the providers of every possible medical effort to save the patient's life. Only when all treatment has failed and the patient is pronounced brain dead is the Organ Bank called.

Inability to Understand Complex Medical Terms and the Unwillingness to Question

Informed consent is a basic tenet of the approach process, and providing it can take more time when probing and explanations are necessary in both English and Spanish. For example, after a long and detailed explanation of brain death and the donation process, one family nodded that they understood what we had discussed, but as soon as I began to walk away, a family member asked another in Spanish, "Is he going to die?" In another situation, an elderly mother from the interior of Mexico was very willing to donate one kidney but reluctant to donate the other, "as he might need it later." When I talked with her further and probed for her understanding of her son's prognosis, it was obvious that she had not understood the physician's explanation of brain death. Hispanic families of lower socioeconomic status are less likely to question directly or admit that they are not completely sure of what is being explained to them.

Strategy

I explain difficult terminology and technical terms as simply as possible. In many cases, I preface my conversation by stating that many people have difficulty with certain words and terms and that I will explain as I go along; if they do not understand, they should stop me and ask me to be clearer. In cases in which I feel that the family is still unsure or unable to understand brain death, I do not pursue the donation option.

Group Decision Making by a Large Extended Family

Ideally, we are told to separate the decision makers from the rest of the family when approaching for donation. With a large extended Hispanic family, it can be difficult to identify the key decision makers (see Chapter 1 of this book). In many cases, every member of the family wants and needs to be involved in the decision-making process. Separating family members from perceived decision makers because we assume that they do not play an important role in family dynamics can cause distrust and an unwillingness to talk and may even anger the family.

Strategy

I anticipate that providing information to a large group will take a great deal of time. I try to encourage every member of the group to ask questions and express their concerns. I believe that consensus is almost mandatory.

Financial Considerations

Many of the families I speak with have basic questions concerning their financial responsibilities, such as "How do I pay the hospital bill?" "How do I get my mother's body from here to Chihuahua?" and "How much will you pay me for her organs?"

Strategy

I try to address all of these questions clearly before consent is requested and obtained. This way, the family members do not feel that they are being rushed into a decision that they do not completely understand nor expect some compensation for their donation.

The Grieving Process

I have found that nurses, because of lack of training, were not very sensitive to Hispanic families because they thought they were too hysterical and distraught to be approached for organ donation. In general, even nurses who have positive feelings about donating organs and tissues believe that the families of potential donors would feel differently and are hesitant to intrude on the family's grief (Vrtis & Nicely, 1993). These families can be approached, but it takes a little more time than usual and requires a larger emotional commitment on the part of the requester. A clear understanding of their support and grieving systems is an essential, if not fundamental, component. Hispanic families are generally more emotionally demonstrative; they hug and kiss acquaintances when greeting them. Children are taught that it is rude not to hug and kiss family members when saying hello or goodbye.

Strategy

Touch has become an important tool when I talk to families; sometimes, something as simple as patting the back of someone's hand can calm a family member enough so that he or she can focus on the most salient issues. This physical contact is not limited by gender. The El Paso staff has added a male Hispanic coordinator who also feels very comfortable approaching grieving families in this way. When Hispanic families are approached in a familiar and thus nonthreatening manner, informed consent becomes more possible because the families can more easily assimilate the information that is given to them.

Sensitivity

The key is to be sensitive to each family's individual needs in the context of their culture. Just as we are very careful to fulfill our agenda when approaching families, pursuing medical history and social history, we need to be sure that we commit the time and effort to fulfill their agenda as well. In my experience, Hispanic families still harbor some mystical feelings about the eyes of their loved one. They will need their eyes to see God or to see other family members who have predeceased them. When Hispanic families are provided with all the information required for true informed consent, in case after case, they have given generously, except for the eyes.

I believe that families, regardless of race or ethnicity, who are given all the information they need will give to their level of understanding. A young couple from Juárez, Mexico, were involved in a motor vehicle accident in El Paso. The couple's 13-month-old daughter was riding unrestrained in the mother's lap. The couple were virtually unhurt, but the child was thrown into the windshield and sustained a head injury that she did not survive. After I had spent a couple of hours with them talking about brain death and organ donation, they decided that they wanted to donate their daughter's heart. They were not sure what all the other organs did, although I did try to give them some basic explanations of the functions of the other transplantable organs. To this young couple with minimal education, the heart was what kept people alive. They wanted to be able to save another child, and they knew their daughter's heart could do that.

Strategy

I try to listen carefully to identify the range of concerns that the family may have regarding the family member in general and the organ donation decision in particular. I make reference to these concerns to emphasize my interest in the general family welfare. I try to accommodate any special requests they may have, such as viewing the body after the surgical recovery. If there are any support services that can help them with the cost and coordination of the transport of the body, I try to make sure that they make contact with the appropriate person within the hospital who can help them.

Language

The crucial barrier for many of the families approached in El Paso is language. Regardless of the family's background, ethnicity, or socio-economic status, you must be able to communicate with them. In El Paso, the Hispanic majority is reflected among its medical professionals at every level. There is no shortage of interpreters. The inability to obtain consent through an interpreter is, I believe, due to the level of training, awareness, and willingness of the interpreter. More important, the requester has a very short time in which to establish trust and rapport with the family, and the individual method that each of us uses does not necessarily come across as intended when our speech is filtered through an interpreter.

Strategy

I do not advocate the use of interpreters, I know that this can be hard for organ banks that do not have a good source of qualified bilingual professionals. But I do not think that you can be successful using an interpreter. Think about watching a foreign film. The actor on the screen says, *"Querida, eres mi cielo, mi mundo, te adoro, te amo,"* which is translated as "I love you." Clearly, something is missed in that translation. All of us put a little of our own personality into the way we approach family. We are trained for that purpose and therefore have learned how to word things in a certain way and have learned how to react to family questions and concerns. The availability of personnel who can discuss the option of organ donation with Spanish-speaking families *in Spanish* and are trained for that purpose made a difference in El Paso. By 1993, 8 out of 20 of the donor families were approached entirely in Spanish.

Outcomes

In 1993, Hispanics accounted for 17 of the 20 total donors. In that same year, 49 of the 60 total referrals received by the organ bank in El Paso were patients of Hispanic origin, and overall, donors had increased from 4 in 1991 to 20 in 1993. The percentage of Hispanic donors rose from 25% in 1991 to 89% in 1993. This increase in Hispanic donors now more accurately reflects the community we serve. More important, the consent rate among this group is beginning to increase as well, from 5.5% in 1991 to 35% in 1993.

By 1996, the consent rate among Hispanics in El Paso had risen to 44%, and the overall consent rate, including non-Hispanics, was 69%. As we continue to address the special needs and language barriers present in our community, we expect to see an even larger increase in Hispanic consent rates. In El Paso, an increase in the Hispanic consent rate translates into a significant increase in total donors.

References

Callender, C. O., Bey, A. S., Miles, P. V., & Yeager, C. L. (1995). A national minority organ/tissue transplant education program: The first step in the evolution of a national minority strategy and minority transplant equity in the USA. *Transplantation Proceedings, 27,* 1441-1443.

Gallup Organization. (1993). *The American public's attitudes toward organ donation and transplantation.* Boston: Partnership for Organ Donation.

Renee, A. A., Viera, E., Daniels, D., & Santos, Y. (1994). Organ donation in the Hispanic population: Donde estan ellos? *Journal of the National Medical Association, 86,* 13-16.

U.S. Bureau of the Census. (1990). *1990 census of population.* Washington, DC: Government Printing Office.

Vrtis, M., & Nicely, B. (1993). Nursing knowledge and attitudes toward organ donation. *Journal of Transplant Coordination, 3,* 70-79.

Chapter 3

PSYCHOLOGICAL RISK FACTORS AND SUBSTANCE ABUSE AMONG YOUNG ADULTS

A Comparison of Non-Hispanic Whites and Mexican Americans

PATRICIA A. LAWRENCE

A survey of 243 undergraduates assessed levels of alcohol and other drug use among Hispanics on the U.S.-Mexico border. It also examined the relationship of substance use to selected social risk factors—problems among family members and use by friends and siblings—and to psychological risk factors—students' sensation- and novelty-seeking needs and stress related to the number of hours students were employed. T tests revealed that beer, wine, hard liquor, and marijuana use are higher among Hispanics whose friends use drugs; wine use is higher if siblings use drugs; but no substance use is higher when family problems exist. Correlation coefficients revealed that beer drinking is higher among students who are employed more than 20 hours per week and that alcohol use is related positively to sensation-seeking needs but negatively to needs for cognitive novelty. Implications for drug prevention strategies are discussed.

The border environment in El Paso, Texas, poses a major threat to the health of its residents—a high risk of illicit substance abuse. El Paso and its "sister city" in Mexico, Juárez, are separated only by a narrow, shallow stretch of the Rio Grande. Three international bridges offer easy entry into either country from the other for almost 100,000 people every day ("Reasons to Cross," 1996). They also facilitate the relatively easy transport of heroin, cocaine, and marijuana into the United States from countries south of the border, consequently flooding the streets of El Paso with cheap, easy-to-buy drugs ("Heroin Flow," 1995). In fact, the El Paso-Ciudad Juárez connection is one of the top three smuggling points for all types of illicit drugs coming into the United States from Mexican and Colombian drug cartels, and federal officials say they know that the largest drug-smuggling organizations in Mexico use the El Paso-Ciudad Juárez drug corridor to smuggle illegal drugs into the United States, especially cocaine ("FBI Links," 1996; "Summit on Border," 1996; "Summit Should Aid," 1996). Due to these threats to the health of U.S. citizens, El Paso has become a focal point for the Clinton administration's antidrug efforts ("FBI Chief," 1996).

In addition to the abundance of illicit drugs, alcoholic substances are easily available to young people in El Paso. Because the legal drinking age in Juárez is only 18, El Paso teenagers who are too young to purchase beer and liquor in Texas can walk or drive across one of the international bridges and buy either ("El Paso/Juárez Drinking," 1996). Or they can go to one of the many Juárez bars that cater to young people with the come-on "Drink till you drop for only five dollars." These nights of binge drinking—the consumption of five or more drinks at one sitting—can impair judgment and physical performance and have led to violent, bloody confrontations and traffic accidents for many El Paso youth ("Binge Drinking," 1996). There is little doubt that many underage young people take advantage of the opportunity to go to Juárez to drink; a recent survey of 710 high school seniors in El Paso revealed that an alarming 88% of males and 83% of females are already drinking alcohol ("Report," 1996).

Finally, many psychotropic drugs, such as Valium, Prozac, and Rohypnol, can be purchased easily and cheaply in Juárez *farmacias* without a doctor's prescription. Even though this is an illegal activity, according to a youth counselor at one of El Paso's drug rehabilitation agencies, it is a common practice among many El Paso residents (M. Manzo, personal communication, September 14, 1995), and it increases their risks for addiction to mind-altering drugs.

In addition to these environmental factors posed by El Paso's location, some young people on the U.S.-Mexico border may be at even higher risk for substance abuse than others due to the same social and psychological factors that are known to lead to early onset and use of multiple substances by young people in other parts of the country and the world. These include social factors such as problems with family members and substance use by family and friends and psychological factors such as stress brought on by long working hours and a personality trait known as sensation or novelty seeking (Donohew, Palmgreen, & Lorch, 1994; Horvath & Zuckerman, 1992; Hughes, 1993; "Study Links," 1993). This study was designed to investigate those specific etiological factors among Hispanic (Mexican American) young adults in El Paso.

Because little is known about substance abuse rates among Hispanics in terms of these social and psychological risk factors, there appeared to be a need for such a study. Even though this investigation was exploratory, it was based on the expectation that if an understanding of the relationship between these etiological factors and substance use could be revealed, then prevention messages could be strategically designed to reach at-risk Hispanic target audiences. Several studies in other parts of the United States have already verified that proposition (e.g., Cook, 1988; Cook, Helm, & Donohew, 1988; Donohew, 1990; Donohew, Helm, Lawrence, & Shatzer, 1990; Donohew, Lorch, & Palmgreen, 1991; Donohew et al., 1994; Lorch et al., 1994; Palmgreen et al., 1991, 1995). However, all of those studies were conducted on non-Hispanic populations living in cities far removed from the U.S.-Mexico border.

Some studies on alcohol and other kinds of substance abuse among Mexican Americans have revealed risk factors that are primarily socioeconomic or culturally based, such as high school dropout rates (Marin, Posner, & Kinyon, 1993); high poverty levels (Harrison & Kennedy, 1994); early onset of substance use, leading to poor cognitive abilities and management skills (Simpson & Barrett, 1991); drinking habits formed before entering the United States (Gilbert & Cervantes, 1986); and tolerance for social deviance, especially alcohol consumption (Casavantes, 1976). Yet none of those studies identified or examined the factors of interest here, all of which are explained below.

Psychological Risk Factors

Employment-Related Stress

Students who hold down jobs are at higher risk for alcohol consumption than are those who are unemployed. Evidence that the number of hours worked and students' levels of alcohol use are positively linked emerged in a study of 1,800 high school students ("Study Links," 1993). Employment while attending school apparently not only provides money to buy drugs but also imposes added stress on students, according to that study. Because many Hispanic students work while attending college, often to supplement their families' income, this factor may affect their levels of alcohol and other substance use; thus, it was examined here.

Sensation and Novelty Seeking

Sensation and novelty seeking are psychological traits that predispose people either to look for or to avoid exciting and unusual people, places, and activities (Pearson, 1970, 1971; Zuckerman, 1979, 1983). High sensation seekers are almost always on the lookout for excitement; they act impulsively, tend to be unconventional, take more risks than average individuals, and eagerly approach new and/or dangerous activities. For example, high sensation seekers like to ride roller coasters, go skydiving, and meet and mingle with unconventional people; they also get bored easily when things rarely change. Conversely, low sensation seekers have a low tolerance for novelty; they tend to shy away from the unusual because they prefer events and situations that are familiar, nonthreatening, and comfortable. These people are content with routines; they are not apt to try new foods or take trips without first making careful plans, and they do not get bored being around the same people every day. Of particular importance is that high sensation seekers are much more likely to abuse alcohol and other drugs than are low sensation seekers.

Sensation- and novelty-seeking tendencies can be measured with self-administered questionnaires; these instruments contain a list of activities and ask respondents to indicate those that appeal to them. The Sensation-Seeking Scale measures four dimensions of the trait: (a) *thrill and adventure seeking*—a tendency to seek out physically risky activities; (b) *experience seeking*—a tendency to prefer nonconforming lifestyles, travel, music, art, drug use, and unconventional friends; (c) *disinhibition*—a need for social stimulation through parties, social drinking, and a variety of sex partners; and (d) *boredom susceptibility*—an aversion to boredom brought on by unchanging conditions or people (Zuckerman, 1979; Zuckerman, Kolin, Price, & Zoob, 1964). The Novelty-Seeking Scale also measures four dimensions of the trait: (a) *external sensation*—a preference for exciting physical activities; (b) *internal sensation*—a need to experience unusual internal feelings; (c) *external cognitive novelty*—stimulation brought on by solving puzzles, planning moves in checkers or chess, and taking things apart and putting them back together; and (d) *internal cognitive novelty*—pleasure brought on by daydreaming, fantasizing, and thinking about why people act the way they do (Pearson, 1970, 1971).

Both scales have been used to weigh the effects of sensation and novelty seeking on responses to mass media and drug prevention campaigns (cited above). Those studies have provided ample evidence that both high and low sensation seekers can be reached with prevention strategies that feature elements that appeal to one group or the other. In addition, the eight subscales have consistently been shown to be highly reliable, with Cronbach alphas ranging from .63 to .89 in a variety of studies (e.g., Cook et al., 1988; Donohew et al., 1990, 1991, 1994; Donohew, Palmgreen, & Rayburn, 1987; Lawrence & Palmgreen, 1991, 1996). Thus, it has been shown that if designers of health prevention campaigns know the psychographic makeup of their target audiences, the chances of preventing or reducing substance abuse among those populations are increased. However, at the present time, there is a void in the literature regarding the existence of these psychological risk factors among Hispanics in the United States.

The Present Study

This study tested the significance of the relationship between drug use and family-related problems among young adult Hispanics, while acknowledging that no one currently knows which condition precedes the other. It also examined the concept of peer pressure by assessing levels of personal substance use by siblings' and friends' use. It further tested the effects of certain psychological risk factors on alcohol and other drug use by examining the strength of the relationship between use and students' tendencies to engage in sensation- and novelty-seeking behaviors and the number of hours that Hispanic students work while enrolled in college. In so doing, the study attempted to provide a social and psychographic profile of young adult Hispanics in terms of those potential risk factors.

Methodology

This study used a survey methodology; it was conducted at the University of Texas at El Paso (UTEP), the largest minority institution (64.4% Hispanic) in the United States, which is located on the U.S.-Mexico border. The survey was funded by a University Research Institute grant.

Subjects

A sample of 243 undergraduates, enrolled in 10 sections of a basic public speaking course, SPCH 3101, completed self-administered questionnaires. SPCH 3101 is a required course for all liberal arts majors at UTEP; thus, the sample was deemed representative of that student population. Students received bonus points toward their "participation grade." However, because that grade accounted for only 5% of their total points accumulated over the course of the semester, participation in the survey had a minimal effect on students' grades. A cover letter, attached to the questionnaire, promised complete anonymity, and although participation was voluntary, all students present on the data collection days completed questionnaires.

Instruments

The questionnaire was designed to provide a demographic and psychographic profile of the students in terms of the variables of interest. Demographic items included sex, age, ethnic group, and number of hours worked per week. Drug use was measured by asking students to indicate how often they currently used cigarettes, beer, wine/wine coolers, marijuana, hard liquor, cocaine, heroin, tranquilizers, and amphetamines; this section of the questionnaire used 6-point Likert-type scales on which 0 indicated *never* and 6 indicated *several times a day*. Students also were asked to indicate the age at which they first used each of those drugs and all the contexts in which they would be most likely to use them: for example, when alone or with friends and when feeling happy or sad. To assess future substance use, respondents were asked to put a check mark next to all the drugs they would probably use in the next 30 days. The substances were listed again, and respondents were asked to answer "yes" or "no" to the question "Do any of your *close* friends or siblings (brothers or sisters) use the drugs listed below?" To test the influence of parental presence on substance use, respondents were asked to respond "yes" or "no" if they still lived at home with their parents. To test the impact of family problems, students were asked to answer "yes" or "no" to the statement "Many family members have problems getting along with each other. Does your family

have this problem?" Sensation-seeking tendencies were measured by listing the 40 activities[1] in Zuckerman et al.'s (1964) scale and asking students
to "indicate how much each statement sounds like you" on 5-point Likert-
type scales on which 1 indicated *this doesn't sound like me at all* and 5
indicated *this sounds exactly like me.* Novelty seeking was assessed by
listing 20 items[2] from Pearson's (1970, 1971) 80-item scale and asking
students to "indicate how much you like or would like to do each activity"
on 5-point Likert-type scales on which 1 indicated *I definitely do not/would
not like to do this* and 5 indicated *I definitely do/would like to do this.* In
both scales, subscale items were randomly ordered to reduce response bias.
A space was provided at the end of the questionnaire for any comments
that students wanted to make.

Statistical Analysis

All data were analyzed using SPSS-X (SPSS, 1988). Summative
scores were computed for the total Sensation- and Novelty-Seeking Scales
and for each of the eight subscale scores. Frequencies were run to determine
the number of students who currently were using various substances.
Correlations between use of one drug with other drugs, between use and
sensation/novelty seeking, and between use and number of hours worked
were assessed with Pearson zero-order correlation tests. Frequencies were
run on the summative sensation/novelty-seeking scores, and after the
median was determined, the total sample was split into high and low
sensation seekers. Cross-tabulations with chi-square tests of independence
were then conducted to test the likelihood that drug use was influenced by
these psychological risk factors by ethnic group. Then, for Hispanics only,
partial correlations, controlling for age, were run to test the relationship
between sensation/novelty-seeking needs and use of various substances,
and two-tailed *t* tests were conducted to examine differences in drug use
levels by sex, substance use by friends and siblings, respondents' place of
residence (at home with parents or not with parents), and presence or
absence of family problems.

Results

The demographic makeup of the full sample closely reflected that of the
student population at the university: A clear majority (63.8%) were His-

panic, 27.2% were non-Hispanic white, 4.9% were African American, 2.1% were Native American, and 1.8% were "other." The sample contained more females (57.6%, *n* = 140) than males (42.4%, *n* = 103). Students' ages ranged from 17 to 58, but most (81%) were younger than 24 (*M* = 22.3; *Mdn* = 20; mode = 19). Most (75.3%) were full-time students carrying academic loads of 12 or more hours. Over half (59.1%) of the full sample, including 58.7% of the Hispanic students, were employed; 33.7% of all, including 32.3% of the Hispanic, working students said that they worked more than 20 hours per week. A clear majority (71%) of the students still lived at home with their parents, but Hispanics outnumbered non-Hispanics by a margin of 78.7% to 57% (χ^2 = 12.68; *p* < .001) on that measure.

Alcohol and Other Substance Use

Well over half of the respondents reported that they currently were using alcohol in one form or another, and there were no statistically significant differences in use levels between Hispanics and other ethnic groups on these measures. For all students, wine/wine coolers use was the highest (72.1%), closely followed by beer (71.2%) and then hard liquor (52.3%). Slightly more than one fifth (22.2%) of the full sample reported that they smoke cigarettes, a finding similar to that for marijuana use (21.4%). Hispanic students reported slightly higher use of cocaine (3.2%) and tranquilizers (4.5%) than did non-Hispanics (1.2% and 2.3% respectively), but lower use of amphetamines (1.3% to 2.3%). No students reported current use of heroin (see Table 3.1). Frequency of use for all drugs was relatively low overall, and no differences emerged in *t* tests comparing Hispanics to non-Hispanics on any of those measures. For example, the average use rates (means) for various substances within the two groups, respectively, were as follows: cigarettes (2.12 to 2.80), wine/wine coolers (2.15 to 2.23), beer (2.51 to 2.60), hard liquor (1.92 to 2.02), marijuana (1.81 to 1.95), cocaine (1.60 to 2.0), tranquilizers (2.71 to 2.0), and amphetamines (1.5 to 1.33). Thus, although many students were using drugs, primarily alcoholic beverages, they reported using them infrequently: that is, less than once a month.

Onset of Drug Use

About one fourth (26%) of all the students currently using various substances reported that they had first used them when they were 12 to 14

TABLE 3.1 Percentages of Substance Abuse by Ethnic Group

Substance	All N = 243	Hispanic n = 155	non-Hispanic n = 88
Wine/wine coolers	72.1	72.8	69.3
Beer	71.2	69.5	74.0
Hard liquor	52.3	50.6	54.5
Cigarettes	22.2	22.1	21.6
Marijuana	21.4	20.3	21.6
Tranquilizers	4.1	4.5	2.3
Cocaine	2.9	3.2	1.2
Amphetamines	2.1	1.3	2.3

years old, and about 10% reported that they had drunk beer (9.4%) or hard liquor (9.8%) before the age of 12. No significant differences were found between Hispanics and non-Hispanics. However, among Hispanics, all substances, even those not currently being used, were first used before they graduated from high school: cigarettes (94.0%), beer (93.3%), wine/wine coolers (92.3%), marijuana (93.6%), hard liquor (91.1%), cocaine (60.0%), heroin (50%), tranquilizers (69.2%), and amphetamines (77.8%). Almost all of the alcohol users reported that they had first drunk wine (95.7%), beer (99.2%), or hard liquor (92.2%) before they reached the legal drinking age of 21 (see Table 3.2). Furthermore, at least one fourth of them had used those substances before they reached high school age (26.7%, 34.7%, and 24.4%, respectively). In addition, more cigarette users had first smoked in junior high (38.8%) than in high school (31.3%), and some had smoked as early as elementary school age (22.4%). In comparison, marijuana use had begun more at the high school (46.8%) than at the junior high (34%) or elementary school (4.3%) levels. Yet before they had graduated from high school, 93.6% of the marijuana users were already using that drug. Among the few Hispanic cocaine users (n = 15), most (53.3%) had first used the drug while in high school, and one third (33.3%) had started using it after they graduated. Thus, the data clearly revealed that most Hispanic alcohol users had begun drinking long before reaching the legal age of 21. In addition, they had started smoking cigarettes before the legal age of 18, and onset of marijuana use peaked during high school. Cocaine use followed the same pattern, with fewer students starting to use that drug after

TABLE 3.2 Onset/Age at Which Hispanic Substance Users First Used Various Drugs

Substance	Age 6-11	12-14	15-18	19-20	21+	n
Wine/wine coolers	3.4%	23.3%	62.1%	3.4%	4.3%	116
Beer	4.2%	30.5%	57.6%	5.9%	0.8%	118
Hard liquor	4.4%	20.0%	65.6%	1.1%	7.8%	90
Cigarettes	22.4%	38.8%	31.3%	4.5%	1.5%	67
Marijuana	4.3%	34.0%	46.8%	2.1%	4.3%	47
Cocaine	0	6.7%	53.3%	33.3%	6.7%	15

high school graduation or after reaching age 21 than while attending high school.

Contexts for Substance Use

Of the total group of current wine/wine cooler and beer users, almost all (95.7%) reported that they drank either when they were with other people (74.5%) or when they were feeling good/happy (21.2%). A similar finding emerged for other alcohol use, with 92.4% of current hard liquor users indicating that they drank when they were socializing (72.6%) or feeling happy (19.8%). A few (8.1%) of the Hispanics, and 2.8% of the non-Hispanic whites, reported that they currently drank hard liquor when they were feeling sad or depressed. In addition, 8.8% of the female current users of hard liquor reported that they drank when they felt sad or depressed, compared to only 3.8% of male drinkers.

Almost all (82.5%) of the marijuana users said that they smoked pot when they were with other people (70%) or when they were happy (12.5%). Of the remaining few, 15% said they used the drug when they were alone; approximately the same percentages were found among Hispanics (14.3%) as among non-Hispanics (12.5%), and for all respondents, slightly more females (16.7%) than males (13%) reported using marijuana when they were alone. Of the small number of cocaine users (2.9%), all reported that they used that drug when they were with other people or when they felt happy; there were no differences by ethnic group or by sex. Among the tranquilizer users, one third said they used these drugs when they were socializing or feeling happy; all were Hispanics and were predominantly males. Another third were non-Hispanic females who reported that they used tranquilizers when they were alone. The remaining third were Hispanic females who used tranquilizers when they were sad or depressed. Close to half (42.9%) of the total number of amphetamine users said that they used these drugs when they were with other people; all were non-Hispanic whites, with a 2:1 ratio of females to males. All of those who said that they used amphetamines when they were happy or alone were female non-Hispanics, and one Hispanic male said that he used amphetamines when he felt sad or depressed.

Multiple use of various substances by Hispanics was revealed in a correlation matrix that examined the relationship of use of each drug to all others. Beer use was positively and significantly related to use of four other substances: wine/wine coolers ($r = .37, p < .01$), hard liquor ($r = .37, p < .01$), cocaine ($r = .91, p < .001$), and marijuana ($r = .47, p < .05$). Use of wine/wine coolers also was positively and significantly related to hard liquor use ($r = .39, p < .01$). Beer consumption was positively related to the number of hours that students worked ($r = .19, p < .05$), suggesting that the more hours that Hispanic students work, the more likely they are to drink beer. Two-tailed t tests revealed three differences between male and female Hispanics in terms of their substance use. Males reported significantly higher rates than did females for use of beer ($t = 2.77, p < .01$) and marijuana ($t = 3.09, p < .01$), but females reported somewhat higher use of wine/wine coolers ($t = 1.09, p = .061$).

Social Risk Factors

Among Hispanics only, the following percentages said that they had close friends who used substances: cigarettes, 67.7%; beer, 92.9%; wine/wine coolers, 93.5%; marijuana, 40.6%; hard liquor, 66.5%; cocaine, 12.9%; heroin, 3.9%; amphetamines, 6.5%; and tranquilizers, 7.7%. These figures were considerably higher than reported substance use among respondents' brothers and sisters: cigarettes, 23.5%; beer, 61.8%; wine/wine coolers, 57.9%; marijuana, 11.9%; hard liquor, 25.8%; cocaine, 2.6%; heroin, none; amphetamines, 2.0%; and tranquilizers, 4.0%.

Two-tailed t tests revealed that Hispanics whose siblings used various drugs did not themselves use substances at higher levels than did those whose siblings did not use drugs. An exception occurred for heavier wine/wine coolers use if siblings drank wine ($t = 2.25$, $p < .05$), smoked marijuana ($t = 2.03$, $p < .05$), used tranquilizers ($t = 1.99$, $p < .05$), or smoked cigarettes ($t = 2.93$, $p < .01$). However, many significant differences were found between Hispanics whose friends used drugs and those whose friends did not. Hispanics with friends who smoked cigarettes drank beer more often than those with friends who were nonsmokers ($t = 2.12$, $p < .05$). Those with friends who drank beer or hard liquor reported higher personal levels of hard liquor ($t = 2.21$, $p < .05$) and beer ($t = 2.86$, $p < .01$) use. Beer drinking was also more frequent ($t = 4.64$, $p < .001$) among Hispanics whose friends smoked marijuana. Finally, marijuana use was significantly higher ($t = 2.12$, $p < .05$) among Hispanics whose friends used cocaine than among those whose friends did not. The data suggest that there is a reciprocal relationship between the levels of substance use by friends and personal use. Some Hispanics' drug use behavior may be influenced by their friends' use, or they may seek out and cultivate friendships with others with similar levels of substance use.

Living at home with parents did not affect levels of substance use among the Hispanic respondents; there were no significant differences between those who lived at home and those who did not. In addition, only a little more than one fourth (27%) of the total sample reported that their family members had problems getting along with each other. Slightly fewer (25.3%) of the Hispanic respondents answered "yes" to this question than did non-Hispanics (29.9%), but that difference was not significant. However, in the cross-tabulation by sex, significantly more ($\chi^2 = 10.65$, $p < .01$) females (35.2%) than males (12.1%) reported that their families were experiencing interpersonal problems. Yet *t* tests between males and females revealed no significant differences in use levels for any of the drugs by the presence or absence of family problems. These findings, combined with the context in which respondents said that they used various substances, hint that alcohol and other drug use among Hispanics may be triggered more by socializing with friends who use drugs than by family problems or substance use by siblings. On the other hand, some Hispanics, like non-Hispanics, may have needs for novelty and sensation that predispose them to use drugs (e.g., see studies cited above on sensation seeking and substance use). This interpretation was borne out when respondents' novelty-and sensation-seeking tendencies were analyzed in relation to their substance use.

Psychological Risk Factors

The cross-tabulation analysis revealed that current use of various substances was occurring more frequently among high sensation seekers than among students with lower needs for excitement, regardless of ethnic group (see Table 3.3). In addition, even though the numbers of respondents reporting tranquilizer, cocaine, and amphetamine use were small, all these respondents were high sensation seekers. However, beer and wine use levels were more similar for both high and low sensation seekers than were levels of cigarette, hard liquor, and marijuana use. These findings differed somewhat from those found among substance users from other ethnic groups because they indicated that the majority of Hispanics used beer and wine at fairly high levels, regardless of their sensation-seeking needs. However, they confirmed findings from other studies (cited above) by indicating that high sensation seekers, including Hispanics, are at high psychological risk for use of illicit drugs such as marijuana and cocaine.

A Pearson zero-order correlation matrix was examined to determine which of the Sensation-Seeking Scale's subscale scores were most strongly related to substance use. It included correlation coefficients for the total Sensation-Seeking Scale scores and the subscales: Thrill and Adventure Seeking, Experience Seeking, Need for Disinhibition, and Boredom Susceptibility. The analysis clearly revealed that the subscale scores explain alcohol and marijuana use better than does the full sensation-seeking score (see Table 3.4). More significant relationships occurred between use and Hispanic students' experience-seeking needs and their needs for disinhibition than occurred for their thrill-and-adventure-seeking and boredom susceptibility tendencies. In addition, these significant correlations held when controlling for age. The stronger relationships between substance use and these first two needs, in particular, suggested that Hispanics with higher scores on the experience seeking and disinhibition subscales tend to seek out physically attractive people and that they like to party, do things that are a little dangerous or exciting, dress in any way they want to, and travel and try new foods. All four sensation-seeking needs correlated significantly with beer use, and all but boredom susceptibility related to hard liquor use. Considered together, these findings indicated that Hispanics who use alcohol and marijuana do so to feel good and to satisfy their needs for social stimulation, not necessarily to keep from getting bored or to engage in physically risky activities.

A second correlation matrix examined the relationship of drug use, novelty seeking, and that scale's four subscales: External Sensation Needs,

TABLE 3.3 Percentages of Substance Users by Sensation Seeking
by Ethnic Group

	Sensation-Seeking Tendency			
	Hispanic		Non-Hispanic White	
Substance	High	Low	High	Low
Wine/wine coolers	85.1	67.5	82.9	68.2
Beer	83.6	58.8	82.9	63.6
Hard liquor	70.1	37.5	68.6	45.5
Cigarettes	35.8	12.5	31.4	13.6
Marijuana	34.3	8.8	40.0	4.5

Internal Sensation Needs, External Cognitive Needs, and Internal Cognitive Needs. The matrix revealed that all four subscale scores were significantly and positively related to marijuana use, suggesting that this drug satisfies various novelty-seeking needs. However, when controlling for age, only needs for internal sensation and internal cognitive novelty correlated significantly with marijuana use, suggesting that smoking marijuana satisfies these two needs, regardless of age. Only the needs for internal and external sensation were significantly and positively related to one other substance—hard liquor (see Table 3.5). In other words, students' needs to lose themselves in daydreams and fantasies about, or to actually engage in, novel activities that evoke thrills and chills were the primary needs that were related to use of two substances. Conversely, their needs for both internal and external cognitive novelty were not only weakly but also, in some cases, negatively related to use of tobacco and alcohol. This finding hinted that some Hispanics with high needs for cognitive novelty (i.e., to discover how things work, plan moves in checkers or chess, solve problems, learn how to do new things or take things apart and put them back together, think about new ideas, and figure out why people behave in certain ways) may search for outlets other than drug use to gratify these particular novelty-seeking needs.

Probable Future Use of Drugs

When asked to indicate which drugs they would probably use in the next month, students' intention-to-use percentages were lower than those

TABLE 3.4 Zero-Order Correlations Between Needs for Sensation and Drug Use

Substance	SSS	TAS	ES	DIS	BS
Wine/wine coolers	.23*	.16	.21*	.29**	.05
Beer	.33**	.23*	.26**	.46**	.33**
Hard liquor	.32**	.29**	.28**	.33**	.14
Cigarettes	.13	.07	.14	.13	.03
Marijuana	.22	.19	.53**	.08	.13

NOTE: SSS, total sensation-seeking score; TAS, thrill and adventure-seeking score; ES, experience-seeking score; DIS, need for disinhibition score; BS, boredom susceptibility score.
*$p < .05$. **$p < .01$.

they reported for current use, dropping to 53.6% for wine/wine coolers, 51.9% for beer, 23.2% for hard liquor, 11.4% for cigarettes, 8% for marijuana, 1.3% for cocaine, 3.4% for tranquilizers, and 0.8% for amphetamines. Among Hispanic respondents, two statistically significant differences were found by sex: More males (63.6%) than females (37.1%) said they would probably drink beer ($\chi^2 = 10.70$, $p < .01$), and more males (13.6%) than females (3.4%) indicated that they would use marijuana ($\chi^2 = 5.59$, $p < .05$). Taken as a whole, the differences between future and current use suggested that some current substance users may be thinking about stopping.

Conclusion and Implications

Several findings emerged here that have important implications for health professionals interested in preventing or reducing alcohol and other drug use among Hispanics, especially those living in high-risk border areas. Of particular interest is that the substance users here began using drugs before they graduated from high school. This finding is similar to that by Simpson and Barrett (1991), and it suggests that because of the high prevalence and easy access to a variety of substances in border cities, prevention efforts must be initiated long before students reach high school if they are to be effective (Harrison & Kennedy, 1994).

The high rates of alcohol consumption are important indicators that prevention programs must be targeted in geographical areas where Hispan-

TABLE 3.5   Zero-Order Correlations Between Needs for Novelty
and Drug Use

Substance	NSS	ES	IS	EC	IC
Wine/wine coolers	.03	.13	.07	−.08	.03
Beer	−.02	.12	.07	−.06	−.16
Hard liquor	.11	.22*	.19*	−.04	.05
Cigarettes	.06	.19	−.25	.09	.11
Marijuana	.45*	.25*	.30*	.23*	.34*

NOTE: NSS, total novelty-seeking score; ES, external sensation needs score; IS, internal sensation needs score; EC, external cognitive needs score; IC, internal cognitive needs score.
*$p < .05$.

ics are concentrated, as also suggested by Harrison and Kennedy (1994). Because most students said they drank primarily when they were with other people, the usage rates strongly suggest that Hispanics' experience-seeking and disinhibition needs are satisfied through social drinking. This conclusion seems warranted in light of the positive relationship between those needs and alcohol use, and it is confirmed somewhat by comments written by four respondents on their questionnaires. For example, Hispanic females wrote: "Usually my friends and I like to unwind on the weekends with a couple of beers and maybe some liquor. We aren't really into the heavy drugs. We don't drink all the time, either. We just want to get away after a long week." "I'm for alcohol, but I don't use it every day—just socially. I live with my grandparents, and they smoke and drink. My drinking is also influenced by my friends and other relatives." "Even though some of my friends and I drink sometimes, it is always in moderation. No one has ever gotten out of hand, and we are very responsible. We are not alcoholics. We don't *have* [sic] to drink. We just like the way it tastes." "I am an occasional social drinker. I drink when I go out dancing. I don't drink to get drunk." Yet the high rates of alcohol consumption, combined with the early onset of wine and beer use among the students surveyed here, could still indicate that Hispanics are at high risk for alcohol addiction, especially in light of the fact that some of their needs for psychological sensation/novelty are strongly related to hard liquor use.

The similar rates of cigarette smoking and marijuana use suggest that marijuana may not appeal to nonsmokers. They also suggest that close to one fourth of Hispanics are at high risk for other substance use, especially considering the claim by Marin et al. (1993) that nicotine use by Hispanics may constitute an important gateway drug for use of other substances. More smoking cessation campaigns need to be aimed primarily at Hispanics, in light of the fact that Hispanics smoke more than do non-Hispanics (Marin et al., 1993).

The fact that interpersonal problems within the family do not affect consumption of various drugs is puzzling. It may be that respondents here were reluctant to reveal accurately their levels of substance use due to a social desirability bias often present in survey data. However, it also may be that Hispanic families confront and resolve problems and, by so doing, do not allow conflicts to lead to substance use among family members. Conflict resolution strategies among Hispanic families warrant further investigation; the findings could be extremely helpful for drug prevention strategists.

The low percentages of students who intend to use alcohol and other drugs in the future is encouraging, especially if they indicate that some users have given some thought to stopping. If this is the case, then intervention campaign messages would be likely to have positive effects, especially if they are strategically designed: that is, if they contain high-sensation-value elements that are known to be effective in grabbing and then holding the attention of psychologically at-risk Hispanic target audiences.

The finding that high needs for cognitive novelty are negatively related to substance use strongly suggests that young Hispanics can be prevented from using drugs if they have ample opportunities to learn about, and engage in, mentally challenging activities. A local example lends credence to this suggestion. An 11-year-old Hispanic elementary school student in El Paso, categorized as at risk 2 years ago, recently won a national chess championship in a field of 500 young competitors. His teachers now say he is "a genius," and they credit chess with helping him and other young students improve their math, problem-solving, and critical thinking skills ("Chess Whiz," 1996). Programs such as this could divert young Hispanics away from drug use by satisfying their perhaps overlooked needs for cognitive novelty.

The experience-seeking risk factor could also be satisfied with activities such as opportunities to participate in school plays, field trips, or dance classes, to name a few. El Paso is a poor city, and many Hispanics there do not have money to travel; the city also is so far from other large U.S. cities that it is almost isolated geographically. Offering young Hispanics opportunities to act out new roles could satisfy their needs to meet new people and engage in behaviors that are somewhat unconventional. Sensation-seeking needs peak at puberty (Farley, 1988); thus, it is important to help young people find socially acceptable ways to satisfy them rather than risking the chance that they will experiment with drugs and harm their health.

Limitations

This study included only young adult Hispanics living in a large U.S.-Mexico border city. In that respect, the population studied here may be unique, and the findings may not be generalizable to Hispanics who live in other parts of the United States. Surveys of younger Hispanics, such as elementary and middle school students, and of Hispanics in other geographical areas need to be conducted to investigate these psychological risk factors so that prevention efforts can address those needs.

Conclusion

Taken together, these data provide findings that have far-reaching implications for drug prevention specialists. There is little doubt that socio-economic factors influence substance abuse among Hispanics, but apparently so do the social and psychological factors investigated here, at least among college-age Hispanics. Follow-up studies need to be conducted using younger Hispanics. If the findings hold, perhaps the risks for substance abuse can be addressed before actual use takes hold and, in that way, prevent alcohol and other drug addictions among Hispanic populations, especially those living in high-risk border cities.

Notes

1. Available from the author on request; address to Dr. Patricia A. Lawrence, School of Communication, University of Idaho, 205 Communication Bldg., Moscow, ID 83844-1072, ph. (208) 885-6458/885-2846.
2. Available from the author on request; address to Dr. Patricia A. Lawrence, School of Communication, University of Idaho, 205 Communication Bldg., Moscow, ID 83844-1072, ph. (208) 885-6458/885-2846.

References

Binge drinking. (1996, March 25). *El Paso Herald Post,* p. 1A.

Casavantes, E. (1976). *El Tecato: Social and cultural factors affecting drug use among Chicanos.* Washington: National Coalition of Spanish Speaking Mental Health Organizations.

Chess whiz. (1996, May 8). *El Paso Herald Post,* p. 1D.

Cook, P. L., Helm, D., & Donohew, L. (1988, May). *Psychophysiological responses to marijuana abuse prevention messages from adolescent audiences: Information for designers of public health campaigns.* Paper presented at the meeting of the International Communication Association, Montreal.

Cook, P. L. (1988, April). *Relationships between sensation seeking subscales and illicit drug use among adolescents.* Paper presented at the Alcohol, Drug Abuse, and Mental Health Administration/National Institute of Mental Health Conference on Loss of Self-Regulatory Control: Its Causes and Consequences, Bethesda, MD.

Donohew, L. (1990). Public health campaigns: Individual message strategies and a model. In E. B. Ray & L. Donohew (Eds.), *Communication and health: Systems and applications.* Hillsdale, NJ: Lawrence Erlbaum.

Donohew, L., Helm, D., Lawrence, P., & Shatzer, M. (1990). Sensation seeking, marijuana use, and responses to prevention messages. In R. R. Watson (Ed.), *Prevention and treatment of drug and alcohol abuse* (pp. 73-93). Clifton, NJ: Humana.

Donohew, L., Lorch, E. P., & Palmgreen, P. (1991). Sensation seeking and targeting of televised anti-drug PSAs. In L. Donohew, H. E. Sypher, & W. J. Bukoski (Eds.), *Persuasive communication and drug abuse prevention* (pp. 209-226). Hillsdale, NJ: Lawrence Erlbaum.

Donohew, L., Palmgreen, P., & Lorch, E. P. (1994). Attention, need for sensation, and health communication campaigns. *American Behavioral Scientist, 38,* 310-322.

Donohew, L., Palmgreen, P., & Rayburn, J. (1987). Social and psychological origins of media use: A lifestyle analysis. *Journal of Broadcast and Electronic Media, 31,* 255-278.

El Paso/Juárez drinking connection spreads to other states. (1996, April 4). *University of Texas at El Paso Prospector,* pp. 1, 4.

Farley, F. (1988, April). *Type T theory (thrill-seeking, risk-taking).* Paper presented at the Alcohol, Drug Abuse, and Mental Health Administration/National Institute of Mental Health Conference on Loss of Self-Regulatory Control: Its Causes and Consequences, Bethesda, MD.

FBI chief, Reno to visit El Paso for drug summit. (1996, June 12). *El Paso Times,* p. 1A.

FBI links federales, drug lord. (1996, July 4). *El Paso Times,* p. 1A.

Gilbert, J. M., & Cervantes, R. C. (1986). Patterns and practices of alcohol use among Mexican Americans: A comprehensive review. *Hispanic Journal of Behavioral Sciences, 8,* 1-53.

Harrison, L. D., & Kennedy, N. J. (1994). Drug use in the United States-Mexico border area: Is there an epidemic waiting to happen? *Hispanic Journal of Behavioral Sciences, 13,* 281-295.

Heroin flow hits high tide in El Paso. (1995, September 18). *El Paso Times,* pp. 1A, 2A.

Horvath, P., & Zuckerman, M. (1992). Sensation seeking, risk appraisal, and risky behavior. *Personality and Individual Differences, 14,* 41-52.

Hughes, R. N. (1993). Relationships between sensation seeking and use of caffeine, alcohol and cigarettes by New Zealand university students. *Drug and Alcohol Review, 12,* 169-173.

Lawrence, P. A., & Palmgreen, P. (1991, May). *Arousal needs and gratifications sought from theatrical films.* Paper presented at the annual meeting of the International Communication Association, Montreal.

Lawrence, P. A., & Palmgreen, P. (1996). A uses and gratifications analysis of horror film preference. In J. Weaver & R. Tamborini (Eds.), *Horror films: Current research on audience preferences and reactions* (pp. 161-178). Hillsdale, NJ: Lawrence Erlbaum.

Lorch, E. P., Palmgreen, P., Donohew, L., Helm, D., Baer, S. A., & Desilva, M. U. (1994). Program context, sensation seeking, and attention to televised anti-drug public service announcements. *Human Communication Research, 20,* 390-412.

Marin, G., Posner, S. F., & Kinyon, J. B. (1993). Alcohol expectancies among Hispanics and non-Hispanic whites: Role of drinking status and acculturation. *Hispanic Journal of Behavioral Sciences, 15,* 373-381.

Palmgreen, P., Donohew, L., Lorch, E. P., Rogus, M., Helm, D., & Grant, N. E. (1991). Sensation seeking, message sensation value, and drug use as mediators of PSA effectiveness. *Health Communication, 3,* 217-227.

Palmgreen, P., Lorch, E. P., Donohew, L., Harrington, N. G., Desilva, M., & Helm, D. (1995). Reaching at-risk populations in a mass media drug abuse prevention campaign: Sensation seeking as a targeting variable. *Drugs and Society, 8*(3/4), 29-45.

Pearson, P. (1970). Relationships between global and specified measures of novelty seeking. *Journal of Consulting and Clinical Psychology, 34,* 199-204.

Pearson, P. (1971). Differential relationships of four forms of novelty experiencing. *Journal of Consulting and Clinical Psychology, 37,* 323-330.

Reasons to cross. (1996, July 3). *El Paso Times,* p. 1A.

Report highlights in El Paso. (1996, June 5). *El Paso Times,* p. 4A.

Simpson, D. D., & Barrett, M. E. (1991). Inhalant use by Mexican American youth: An introduction. *Hispanic Journal of Behavioral Sciences, 13,* 246-255.

SPSS, Inc. (1988). *SPSS-X user's guide* (3rd ed.). Chicago: Author.

Study links students' work hours with alcohol, drugs. (1993, March 26). *El Paso Herald Post,* p. B4.

Summit on border seeks drug solution. (1996, June 15). *El Paso Times,* p. 5A.

Summit should aid El Paso drug war. (1996, July 8). *El Paso Times,* p. 1B.

Zuckerman, M. (1979). *Sensation-seeking: Beyond the optimal level of arousal.* Hillsdale, NJ: Lawrence Erlbaum.

Zuckerman, M. (1983). A biological theory of sensation seeking. In M. Zuckerman (Ed.), *Biological bases of sensation seeking, impulsivity, and anxiety* (pp. 37-76). Hillsdale, NJ: Lawrence Erlbaum.

Zuckerman, M., Kolin, E., Price, L., & Zoob, I. (1964). Development of a sensation seeking scale. *Journal of Consulting Psychology, 28,* 477-482.

Chapter 4

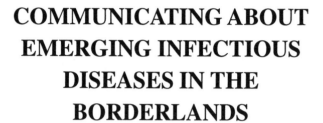

COMMUNICATING ABOUT EMERGING INFECTIOUS DISEASES IN THE BORDERLANDS

Hantavirus Education for Rural, Border, and Migrant Populations

ROBBIN D. CRABTREE
LEIGH ARDEN FORD

In June 1996, the Clinton administration announced plans for a new policy initiative to fight emerging infectious diseases (Manning, 1996). Described as "one of the most significant health and security challenges facing the global community" (p. 1), the infectious diseases of concern included dengue fever, Ebola fever, and hantavirus. In part, this policy initiative is meant to establish global surveillance and response systems and to encourage research on emerging infectious disease.

AUTHORS' NOTE: We wish to acknowledge the collaboration of Dr. Colleen Jonsson, Department of Chemistry and Biochemistry at New Mexico State University. This research was partially funded by a grant from the State of New Mexico Department of Health, Contract No. 96-665-14-009.

One strategy for developing research programs on emerging infectious disease is to create interdisciplinary teams in which the efforts of medical researchers such as biochemists, virologists, physicians, and epidemiologists are complemented by the efforts of information dissemination researchers such as communication and public health education scholars. Currently, we are participating in a small-scale, collaborative, interdisciplinary research project of this type along the U.S.-Mexico border. The project focuses on the identification and prevention of hantavirus pulmonary syndrome (HPS), initially called the Four Corners virus and now commonly referred to as the *sin nombre* virus in the United States.

This chapter presents a field report of that ongoing borderlands study. The purpose of the chapter is to give a brief sketch of the research project with a particular emphasis on the barriers to effective health communication that we have discovered. These barriers include the complexities of working collaboratively across agencies, communities, and disciplines; the difficulties of developing effective and appropriate health education materials for marginalized and at-risk populations; and the ethical and methodological dilemmas encountered when studying these difficult-to-access groups. We hope that our "tales from the field" (Van Maanen, 1988) will suggest directions for future research, as well as for more effective health communication and education practices in the borderlands.

The Hantavirus Research Project

In the following sections, we provide a description of HPS, its cause, its symptoms, and its consequences. The goal is to illuminate the public health and communication issues associated with this infectious disease. We then describe our borderlands hantavirus identification and prevention research project. We include a description of the research team, the project's goals, and the research strategies employed.

Hantavirus as an Infectious Agent

Hantavirus is the name for a family of viruses thought to have originated in Europe and Asia. This family of viruses is responsible for serious, often life-threatening infections throughout the world. The hantavirus is spread to humans by infected rodents. When the fresh or dried rodent urine or feces shed the virus, it becomes airborne, and the aerosolized virus is inhaled by the human host (Centers for Disease Control and Prevention [CDC], 1994). The infection may also be spread through rodent bites, although such occurrences are rare. Common known vectors of the hantavirus in the United States are the deer mouse and cotton rat (CDC, 1994; Kreeger, 1994). It is important to emphasize here that the hantavirus is not spread through human-to-human contact.

Outbreaks of hantavirus infection in the United States were virtually unknown until the summer of 1993. At that time, several deaths due to severe infection in the lungs were reported in the Four Corners region (Arizona, Colorado, New Mexico, Utah) of the United States (Lemonick, 1993; Reckitt & Coleman, 1994a, 1994b, 1995). The medical community identified the infections as HPS, and the CDC began a focused research effort to identify and prevent this emerging infectious disease.

HPS poses a serious public health threat. Approximately 50% of recently documented cases have resulted in death, 10 times the rate associated with the hantavirus-related Korean hemorrhagic fever (Wenzel, 1994). At present, there is no known cure for HPS. As a consequence, early diagnosis and immediate medical attention are critical to preventing fatalities due to HPS. Symptoms of the hantavirus infection resemble those of flulike viruses and include fever, headaches, severe muscle aches, shortness of breath, dry cough, vomiting, and abdominal pain. Unlike the flu, however, in HPS the fever is nonresponsive to medication, and the muscle aches are so severe that movement is nearly impossible (Reckitt & Coleman, 1994a, 1994b, 1995). Significantly, this resemblance of HPS to flu is one of its most dangerous characteristics because it may prevent people from seeking immediate medical attention (Lemonick, 1993).

Although HPS has been difficult to diagnose, has no known cure, and is often fatal, the disease is quite preventable. Simple measures such as eliminating potential food sources for rodents, cleaning food storage and other areas with disinfectant, wearing protective masks and gloves to clean up infested sites, and trapping rodents effectively are recommended by the CDC (CDC, 1994; Reckitt & Coleman, 1994a, 1994b, 1995).

Though hantavirus infection can occur in persons of any age, ethnic, racial, gender, or geographic group, "The current epidemic has disproportionately affected members of minorities living in rural settings" (Wenzel, 1994, p. 1004). Experts feel that those who live or work around food storage areas, barns, fields, or other potential rodent-infested areas are most at risk. The rural populations of southern Doña Ana County, New Mexico, and the migrant and seasonal farmworkers who come here fit this profile. Furthermore, rural, border, and migrant populations are less likely to have access to information about the disease and its prevention and also are less likely to access health care services even when these are available (Kaplan, Alpert, Blodgett, & Gargas, 1989). Hence, rural, border, and migrant populations are particularly at risk for exposure to this infectious agent and possess little ability to prevent exposure and to respond quickly if infected.

Overview of the Borderlands
Hantavirus Research Project

Hantavirus is one of many emerging infectious diseases currently under examination by medical researchers (e.g., Bremner, 1993; Sands, Kioski, & Komatus, 1993). It has also been the focus of public health campaigns, particularly in the Four Corners area (Kreeger, 1994). As members of the only research team working on hantavirus along the U.S.-Mexico border (P. Ettestad, New Mexico Department of Health, personal communication, August 9, 1996), we have been interested in the communication strategies used to disseminate information about this emerging infectious disease to Spanish-speaking rural, border, and migrant populations. This interest is incorporated in a larger interdisciplinary research project in which seroprevalence screening—that is, testing blood for prior exposure to hantaviral agents—is the goal. The interdisciplinary research team includes one biochemist/virologist, several students (graduate and undergraduate) working in her lab, two development/health communication scholars (ourselves), and one communication studies graduate student. At various points, other members of the university community (students, faculty, librarians, etc.) who are interested in the project and fluent in Spanish have become involved at individual research sites.

The project is partially funded by the New Mexico Department of Health from funds allocated by the CDC. A mobile health clinic unit, which is used at some research sites, is funded by a grant to the Border Health Council, a program of the Public Health Division of the New Mexico Department of Health. In addition, a small grant from the El Paso Community Foundation supports the purchase of hantavirus prevention supplies.

The design of the project combines seroprevalence screening with prevention education and assessment of prevention materials. In this design, study participants first complete a basic health status survey that includes identification of activities known to be risk factors in contracting the hantavirus. Then participants have a small amount of blood drawn. This blood screening indicates whether the individual has been exposed to hantavirus. The test results are available by phone approximately 2 weeks later. A positive result simply indicates exposure to the virus, and, of course, the survival of the exposed person. The positive result then can be matched to the health survey to identify the associated risk factor(s) and the possible source of the infection. The seroprevalence study is in progress, and incidence rate results are not yet available.

The second component of the project is the provision of prevention education and the assessment of the education materials. The prevention education materials were developed by Reckitt & Coleman, Inc. (producers of d-CON rodenticide and Lysol brand disinfectant) in cooperation with the CDC. The CDC also has produced a video describing the origins and nature of hantavirus, its symptoms, and recommended prevention measures. These English-language materials were translated into Spanish under the guidance of the CDC, and the resulting Spanish-language materials are the focus of our portion of the research project. Thus, during or after the blood draw, participants read (or have explained orally) prevention education materials. At some sites, the video is shown as well, and a pre- and postviewing questionnaire is administered.

To assess the effectiveness of the Spanish-language education materials, the strategy is to use focus groups and interviews with rural community health workers, people who live in the towns and rural areas on the U.S.-Mexico border, and migrant farmworkers who gather at the El Paso-Ciudad Juárez border crossing for transportation to the fields. As the following discussion and "tales from the field" indicate, we already have confronted many barriers to the research and can expect other barriers to emerge as we continue this work.

Barriers to Health Communication in the Borderlands

Our experiences in the field to date suggest a number of significant, though not insurmountable, barriers to effective and appropriate health communication in the borderlands. Those barriers discussed here are (a) the complexities of working collaboratively across agencies, communities, and disciplines; (b) the difficulties of developing effective and appropriate health education materials for marginalized and at-risk populations; and (c) the ethical and methodological dilemmas encountered when accessing these populations. For each barrier, we describe the key issues and illustrate with examples from our experience.

Barrier 1: The Complexities of
Collaboration and Cooperation

As suggested by the Clinton policy initiative on emerging infectious diseases, cooperation among agencies and, indeed, countries is required to address the threat represented by emerging infectious diseases. Ongoing efforts along the U.S.-Mexico border reflect this demand for cooperation among the multiple interests, both private and public, attempting to meet the health and development needs of this poor, largely rural area. Though collaboration is certainly desirable, the difficulties of sustained cooperation in an environment of scarce resources, conflicting strategies for achieving goals, and differences in agenda complicate that collaboration. Our experience with the hantavirus project has certainly reinforced that view.

It would be nearly impossible to describe fully the myriad agencies and organizations involved in health issues along the U.S.-Mexico border. Some of the interested parties are publicly funded oversight agencies who may also be responsible for distributing resources and granting access, such as federal and state agencies and consortia and international organizations encouraging cross-border cooperation. Others are public or private research institutions, such as universities or private health consulting firms. Others are service providers, such as not-for-profit clinics, for-profit hospitals, and other health care delivery organizations. And, of course, there are the communities themselves (see Wieder & Hartsell, 1996, for a fascinating discussion of the notion of "community" in public health) on both sides of the border, replete with the inherent political, social, and cultural ambiguities of border living. Essentially, these various stakeholders come to the table with both collaborative and competitive instincts. Hence, the politics of dealing with these myriad agencies can be daunting and can function as a very real barrier to successful health communication research.

What is critical to impart here is that working in health communication and education in the region requires both knowledge and diplomacy. An example of these politics at work comes from our first attendance at a binational meeting of representatives from various border health-related agencies. This group meets regularly under the auspices of one border health agency, whose responsibility is ostensibly to oversee and facilitate health development in the border areas. At this meeting, this agency sponsored, and by default gave sanction to, an economic development project masquerading as health-related research. In the guise of doing a "needs assessment" of the elderly in a pair of border towns (one on the U.S.

side and its sister on the Mexico side), some entrepreneurial consultants working for a major retirement community developer presented the results of their analysis of the needs of this community (field notes, October 27, 1995). The rationale and information presented by these consultants struck us as far from persuasive and as culturally insensitive. However, because we were new participants in this group without a clear understanding of the political dynamics, open questioning of the logic by us was inappropriate. Nonetheless, we did speak privately to the border agency director later and expressed our concerns.

This political complexity was further evidenced at another meeting. At this meeting, delays in the establishment of a low-cost primary care clinic in the border towns named above were the focus of a lengthy discussion. The need for such a clinic is great, given the poverty and low health status of the citizens and the great distance to available care facilities. However, the local political and economic interests were in conflict over the establishment of the clinic.

Still a relative newcomer, one of us suggested that the group write a letter of support for the clinic and encourage state officials to advocate for the clinic as well. These suggestions were acknowledged but not accepted as actions the group could or would take. In fact, in private conversation with one of us, the chair of the group stated that the group used to do advocacy work but had moved away from such efforts.

What is interesting is the manner in which these two incidents and the associated agencies converge politically. Several months later, an article in the local paper revealed that the local government of the border town had voted to place a moratorium of 6 months on the community health clinic scheduled for the area to allow the private group described above time to complete a feasibility study for a development project that included a small shopping center, a recreational vehicle park, a health clinic, and a housing project (Foster, 1996). At this point, these poor communities are likely to see the development of a middle-class retirement village before they see a no/low-cost health clinic.

As we learn all the players and stakeholders, we have been made acutely aware of the sensitivity surrounding interagency competition and politics. Given this scenario, we continually ask ourselves to what degree and in what ways we can involve ourselves in the politics of border health. As we gain more experience, our involvement in such matters is likely to increase as well.

The process of collaboration across the academic disciplines has also produced complexities. As previously mentioned, our team of academics consists of two primary fields of study: biochemistry and communication. As members of different academic communities, we bring different languages, meaning, and worldviews to this project, as well as different goals and methodologies. We have discovered that we have vastly different ways of working, clearly distinct priorities, and remarkably dissimilar professional expectations. Although this combination of expertise has resulted in a very creative collaboration, it has also resulted in a kind of "trained communication incapacity" from which problems in that collaboration arise.

We have found, for example, that whereas drawing blood and examining it in the lab is a precise exercise, assessing education materials cannot be done with a hypodermic needle, as early theories about the impact of communication suggested (see, e.g., Korzenny & Ting-Toomey, 1992; Nair & White, 1993; Severin & Tankard, 1992; Windahl & Signitzer, 1992). For natural scientists, rigor and "good work" derives from a carefully controlled experimental environment in the field and in the laboratory. For us, valid questionnaire design, interview skills, and sensitivity to cultural and contextual factors as well as to power dynamics exemplify rigor and "good work." This means that we prefer to go slower in the field, taking plenty of time to case the scene, gain entry and trust, and respond to cultural differences.

We also had to spend a great deal of time learning about each other's disciplines. For example, we quickly discovered that survey and interview techniques are standard skills for communication scholars but are known to biochemists mainly from reading social research. Further, the research methods of each discipline have their own language and mystique. For example, the statistical analysis of data may use similar terminology but is conducted and understood in differing ways. Finally, working together effectively in interdisciplinary teams means being clear about what is expected of us professionally for tenure and promotion. For instance, obtaining grants is absolutely crucial in biochemistry; hence, the work is driven by the ability to acquire such resources. In communication studies, grants are desirable but by no means required. Here the work is driven by the ability to gain access to persons and their communication behaviors. All these differences can lead to conflicts in priorities and project-related goals and activities.

Although these barriers to collaboration exist, it must be noted that interagency and interdisciplinary cooperation yields rich rewards (Howe-Murphy, Ross, Tseng, & Hartwig, 1989). In a world of ever-shrinking resources, collaboration among agencies and the reduction of duplicate efforts are demanded. Further, and more important, we are able to tackle so much more of the problem (in this case, emerging infectious disease prevention) with a multiple-perspective approach. We are able to learn more about the "big picture" of health communication when we see the scientific and political constraints operating. In addition, granting agencies are increasingly interested in projects that are interdisciplinary in nature and that cooperate with local/community/grassroots efforts. These advantages far outweigh the obstacles.

Barrier 2: Difficulties in Development
of Educational Materials

Effective health communication campaigns begin with careful analysis of the target audience (Lefebvre et al., 1995; Ratzan, Payne, & Massett, 1994; Witte, 1995). For example, the culture, language, salient belief structures, and economic conditions of the targeted population are only a few of the audience characteristics that need to be understood if the information and prevention strategies suggested by an education and prevention campaign are to be adopted by the message recipients (Witte, 1995). The preliminary stages of this study revealed several significant shortcomings in the available Spanish-language hantavirus education materials. These shortcomings illustrate an insufficient understanding of the targeted population that created barriers to successful information dissemination about hantavirus in the borderlands.

The first barrier we encountered resulted from assumptions we had made about the present knowledge level of the participants. We had failed to account for the meaning of *virus* to a population whose access to health-related information is limited. The word *virus* seems to strike a negative chord in people and is currently associated primarily with sexually transmitted diseases (STDs). Indeed, the few surveys we have managed to collect indicate that before viewing the video, people think hantavirus is a sexually transmitted disease.[1] The following illustrates that confusion and our possible contribution to its continuance.

At health fairs, primary education and data collection sites for us, we found that people would often pass by our booth without even making eye contact. Given the sensitive nature of STDs, it is not surprising that people were reluctant to participate in the study if they believed that it was STD related. Further, when persons at health fairs did agree to participate, we frequently found it necessary to explain that hantavirus was not the same as HIV or other viruses that were sexually transmitted, for which they may have been seeking a test. In addition, we may have inadvertently contributed to further confusion at one health fair. Because both HIV testing and our hantavirus screening require blood to be drawn, we arranged for a cooperative single blood draw with persons from the Department of Public Health who were conducting HIV testing. In this process, it was evident that several individuals were unclear about the differences in the two types of testing that were being conducted and also about the differences in the diseases themselves, despite efforts to clarify through informed consent, provision of instruction, and discussion of test result procedures.

A similarly confusing message may have inadvertently been sent when we conducted a blood draw and health education for migrants at the Ciudad Juárez-El Paso border crossing (this trip is described fully in the next section). Here, in an effort to "give back" something to those who participated in our project, we had a basket of free condoms available. Some men who did not participate in the blood draw nonetheless picked up the condoms. In retrospect, the "mixing" of the two viruses in the minds of the workers was perhaps inevitable.

A second and perhaps more significant barrier that we confronted concerned the nature of the education materials themselves. Both the written materials and the video presentation were developed for use with a broad, general, English-speaking audience and then were translated into Spanish for use with Spanish-speaking populations. This process demonstrates that insufficient attention was paid to the characteristics of the rural, border, and migrant population targeted.

First, many of the written materials, those created as a public service by the producers of d-CON and Lysol products and those produced by the CDC, are typified by dense content. Brochures and pamphlets feature thick written text with few illustrations. Further, these illustrations are minimally informative and may even be confusing. For illiterate or poorly educated populations, the use of simple, clear diagrams or cartoons would be more effective (Mody, 1991).

The hantavirus prevention video is also problematic for use with rural, border, and migrant populations. The 27-minute documentary is content dense, containing sections on the evolution of the disease, several testimonials by experts and survivors, a nice treatment of the symptoms, in-depth portrayal of the medical procedures necessary to survive the illness, and extensive illustration of prevention measures. The language in use is "high Spanish," or Castillian-style Spanish,[2] with many graphic titles. Rather than using overdubbing techniques in the translation (reducing the volume of the English audio and dubbing in Spanish translation), the producers used Spanish subtitles (only the narration was changed to Spanish; all "expert" or "survivor" testimony was subtitled). The subtitles are also presented in "high Spanish" and move very quickly. We could see that even literate participants would have trouble keeping up with the constantly moving text.

The video also presents a world distant from the lives and experiences of rural, border, and migrant populations. The expert testimony comes from persons associated with the medical research community. The moving testimonials from HPS survivors in the video are all given by middle-class Anglos (with the exception of one Navajo). Finally, the video features scenes from large wheat farms or from the Four Corners region, scenes likely to be unfamiliar to the targeted population.

It is clear that these materials are inappropriate and ineffective for some Spanish-speaking rural, border, and migrant populations who do not have sufficient educational or literacy levels. Further, the representative scenes and images of hantavirus as presented in this video have only minimal links to the day-to-day experiences of border populations. Although the educational materials have been effective in training utility workers, for instance, who may be at risk, we feel they will be very ineffective in reaching the underresourced, underinformed, and marginalized populations along the border. Fortunately, the CDC has been very responsive to our criticisms and concerns. They have agreed to the creation of a new 7-minute video produced specifically for the rural poor in border Spanish. This video can be played in the mobile medical unit (which is equipped with a TV/VCR), in food stamp offices, in local health clinic lobbies, and so forth. It will feature disease identification and prevention only. In addition, the CDC is in the process of identifying Hispanic hantavirus survivors for interviews in the new production. We will assess the effectiveness of these materials as the project continues.

Barrier 3: Dilemmas in Accessing At-Risk
and Marginalized Populations

Perhaps the most significant barrier to health communication about emerging infectious diseases in the borderlands is the problem of accessing the most marginalized, and in this case the most at-risk, populations. This is a concern that has been expressed in much of the literature on multi-cultural health care and intercultural communication (e.g., Geist, 1994;

Ray, 1996). Though access is superficially a methodological problem, it also generates significant ethical dilemmas that the researcher must face. In our work, efforts to gain access have been challenged by efforts to preserve human dignity.

One of the strategies for accessing rural, border, and migrant populations is to attend local community health fairs. These are generally held at community centers or schools in the small rural towns along the border. Organized by local clinics and schools, representatives from local health care agencies set up tables or booths addressing a myriad of health issues. Typically, services such as cholesterol and diabetes screening, basic nutrition information, blood pressure testing, and dental care figure prominently at health fairs. Most of the information is presented in English, although it is also available in Spanish. In this environment, hantavirus screening and prevention education fit well.

Health fairs are highly fluid events, where people move from booth to booth quickly, stopping here and there but rarely doing more than picking up pamphlets as they pass. Because the available CDC video is 27 minutes long, we had difficulty getting anyone to commit the time to complete pre- and postviewing questionnaires and to watch the CDC video.

In short, we decided that health fairs would not be an ideal site to collect data about a 27-minute video, even though it was an excellent site to find the desired population groups in a naturally occurring setting. Thus, at health fairs, we continue with the seroprevalence portion of the study, do much face-to-face education about hantavirus and its prevention, and continue to distribute pamphlets. We also hope to use the new, shorter format video when it is completed. Currently, the educational component has become almost completely a community service aspect of the project, with few data about the effectiveness of the education materials forthcoming.

Health fairs may be a good way to access rural populations in the borderlands, but they do lead to some ethical dilemmas. First, many attend health fairs with specific health issues they wish to address, such as diabetes screening or child immunizations. As noted in the previous section, most of the population has minimal information about hantavirus and hence low interest in the issue. Thus, persuading individuals to participate in the screening without raising undue alarm becomes a challenge. Further, it was clear that some participants, even after the process of informed consent and a brief education provision, still were unclear about just what kind of blood screening had been done and just what the nature of the virus itself was. In the harried atmosphere of a health fair, further explanations are difficult, if not impossible, to give. Thus, lingering concerns in those being tested may be raised unnecessarily.

Access to the male population and migrant workers in particular has been difficult. The community health fairs are largely attended by women and children, so this is a difficult environment from which to recruit male study participants. Though members of migrant families may attend these health fairs, there may be reluctance to participate in studies due to concerns about legal status and so on. In short, alternative access routes must be used.

Access to migrant worker populations is very problematic generally. One cannot go directly to the fields because this creates political and employment problems for the migrants. To reach the migrant farmworkers and to enlist them in the study, we traveled with the New Mexico Department of Health mobile medical unit on an overnight trip to the Ciudad Juárez-El Paso border crossing (from field notes, March 20, 1996). Here, in the early predawn hours, migrant and seasonal farmworkers gather to catch converted school buses or *raiteros* (privately contracted vans) for transportation to the chile, onion, and corn fields of southern New Mexico.

For this trip, our group included several students; the biochemist; the mobile unit, staffed by a physician's assistant and a phlebotomist; one graduate student's husband, who is Paraguayan; and us. Demographically, the team was composed of six women (two Hispanic, three Spanish speaking) and three men (one Spanish speaking Hispanic). We departed campus at 2:00 a.m. and arrived a few blocks from the border crossing at 3:00 a.m. to find a few men already gathering for the buses. By prearrangement, we met up with a woman who is a volunteer labor organizer working with the farmworkers and who was acting as our liaison. While we set up our tables, coffeepot, basket of condoms (our reciprocity on this trip; see previous section), and the medical unit, our liaison chatted informally with the growing number of migrants. As buses and vans arrived, some men went directly onto the buses; others milled around on the sidewalk. The Paraguayan went into the groups of men to try to recruit people. We felt that a Spanish-speaking male would be most effective at this task. Though much of the team is bilingual, we are predominately female and Anglo.

The men were hesitant to participate and very wary of the whole setup. Much curiosity was expressed from a distance, and individual men approached the tables almost like scouts. It was difficult to explain that a positive blood seroprevalence would not stigmatize the participants (unlike, for example, a positive HIV test, and again, the viruses were being confused). Fear of needles was prolific, and it was apparent that these men rarely had contact with medical care services. It was also difficult to convince the men to participate because they had no inherent interest in the project. We gave information and coffee, and many took free condoms, but they could get all of those things without giving blood. For those who decided to participate, there was some wariness about both the consent form (which many signed with an X) and the questionnaire (which was given orally).

Perhaps the most prevalent fear among the farmworkers was that if they participated, they would miss the bus. The buses fill up on a first-come, first-served basis. Once the seats are full, the driver will not accept more people, and those who miss the bus will miss a day of work. The farmworkers were concerned that if they went into the mobile unit to give blood, they would lose a seat on the bus when the driver decided to depart, a departure time that seemed totally arbitrary to us as observers. We tried assuring them we could complete the process in 5 minutes, but many were unconvinced. To accommodate their concerns, we rushed them through the process, which often meant getting data (blood and questionnaire) but being uncertain about how much disease and prevention information actually was imparted. Out of the approximately 150 men who showed up to work that day, we felt lucky to draw 20 blood samples.

This method of accessing the migrant population is a viable option available to our team. We believe that as we continue to visit this site, we will be able to gain more participation. This method of access, however, is also not without its ethical dilemmas. First, the issue of time for participation is problematic. The entire process of health survey, blood draw, and brief education should take between 20 and 25 minutes. During the time when the men appeared to be simply waiting, we felt comfortable recruiting participants. However, the seemingly arbitrary departure of some vehicles created some anxiety among the migrants and fed our concerns as well. Were the men simply reluctant to participate, or were they truly fearful of missing a bus? The level of persuasion to apply was a dilemma that remains unresolved. As far as we know, one man did miss a bus because of his participation, and we were unable to ascertain if he found other transportation that day.

A more troubling ethical dilemma that arose from this method of access was related to the use of the mobile medical unit. Although this was an ideal setup for the gathering of blood samples, it also represented a possible source of medical care and information to several of the men. In a couple of instances, while the physician's assistant was drawing blood, the participant requested medical advice and/or treatment. For example, one worker had a sore leg and asked for help from the physician's assistant. Under the circumstances, the physician's assistant could offer advice but was not equipped to offer treatment. Thus, we struggle with the tensions between our needs as researchers and the enormous health care needs of this marginalized population.

Critical in gaining access to, and building a trusting relationship with, marginalized populations such as the rural poor and the migrant farmworkers is the role of community gatekeepers. Within communities, the *promotoras,* or community health workers, can facilitate the participation of people living in the *colonias,* or small, poor communities that lack basic infrastructures such as electricity, plumbing, and water. Farmworker union leaders and organizers may be of help in gaining migrant participation, but these links have been difficult for our research team to establish. In some cases, local teachers can be of great help and in our project have even assisted with survey administration. Gatekeepers may only agree to help, however, if they feel that the research will be of benefit to the communities.

This leads to concerns about ethics in research generally and in the specific cases noted previously. From the beginning, our team has tried to be sensitive to the needs and constraints of the border populations. There are complex factors weaving together the tapestry of border society—language, social class, occupation, national origin, generation, gender, ethnic identity, and so forth. Although merely studying these populations may eventually benefit them, they have little control over the questions being asked or the use of the knowledge produced from their responses. This creates an imbalanced power relationship between researcher and researched (Brown & Tandon, 1983), which can only undermine their trust and willingness to participate. For us, it has been important to build reciprocity into the research project as much as possible. This has meant participating in health fairs as a community service without collecting any data at all. We have obtained a small grant just to fund the purchase of hantavirus prevention materials (gloves, masks, disinfectant, traps) that can be distributed to the migrants. And we are moving toward a collaborative and participatory research design for ongoing border health and communication research (see, e.g., Chapter 9 of this book). We have had to discourage the prolific media attention that this project attracts to protect our participants (some of whom may have problems with legal immigration status, for example). And in some cases, we have become advocates for health policy that considers the unique needs of rural, border, and migrant populations.

Conclusion

This field report identifies some key issues in border health communication. First, it is essential for researchers to have a working knowledge of the other players and some insights into the politics that guide relationships between them. Collaboration between researchers and agencies/institutions seems vital, but managing collaboration in a productive way is very difficult. Related to this is the process of interdisciplinary collaboration. Working in a team creates unique problems and misunderstandings. However, these collaborations are likely to be more productive in the long run.

Second, the significance of designing education materials that account for the specific characteristics of the targeted population cannot be overestimated. If prevention of hantavirus is the goal, the information provided must be accessible to those populations specifically at risk. Further, the means for the marginalized population to use the information must be incorporated into the research strategy and goals.

Third, accessing marginalized populations presents challenges beyond imagining to the researcher. It requires sensitivity, trustworthiness, and commitment by the researcher. Most of all, it requires a continuous questioning of oneself and one's actions in the pursuit of a research goal. And it requires the ability to abandon those goals when called on.

Although our research is being conducted along one section of the U.S.-Mexico border using one emerging infectious disease as a case study, the experiences of "border crossing" and the barriers to health communication would certainly be relevant to other binational or multinational projects. The setting and the populations are unique, but the issues are quite generalizable to other settings, as well as back to theory.

In terms of communication theory and research, our project makes several contributions, some of which merely reinforce what researchers have been recommending for years. For instance, Everett Rogers's (1995) influential diffusion of innovations theory pointed out the critical role of opinion leaders in the dissemination and adoption of new ideas and practices. By integrating our efforts with those of lay community health workers, we build a collaboration with local opinion leaders who are already charged with affecting the health status of their communities (see Chapter 9 of this book). Further, the issue of homophily has been cited as critical to successful health and development communication efforts (Nair & White, 1993; Rogers, 1995; Windahl & Signitzer, 1992). That is, messages are more effective and more persuasive when the sender shares characteristics with the receiver.

Social marketing provides an alternative theoretical framework to consider in relation to this project (e.g., Jones, 1982). Clearly, our initial findings suggest that disease prevention education strategies need to be targeted to a wider variety of populations, with particular focus on high-risk and hard-to-reach groups. The America Responds to AIDS campaign is an example of social marketing that has employed multiple approaches to essentially the same message (Ratzan et al., 1994). On the basis of our work, it is clear that migrant farmworkers, for example, require specific message strategies and may even rely on different media than other border populations.

In conclusion, we pose the question, "Which are the borders/boundaries?" Although *the borderlands* refers to the area surrounding the U.S.-Mexico border, we have discovered that the "line in the sand" means very little in terms of health needs or health communication strategies. The communities on both sides of the border are largely Spanish speaking and are very much in need of basic health care and information. The more significant borders, it seems, are the boundaries of social class, education, lifestyle, language, interaction styles, and so on, that exist between researchers and subject populations. It is vital for us to maintain a research agenda that includes disadvantaged and difficult-to-study groups if our work is to be relevant to the communities we investigate. Those who produce disease prevention materials need to seriously reconsider their communication strategies if they hope to reach the most disadvantaged, and thus the most at-risk, populations. We propose the use of collaborative, community-based research projects that draw on participatory-action research methodologies (e.g., Brown & Tandon, 1983; Hall, 1981; Tandon, 1981) and feature strong interagency and community collaborations. After all, the purpose of the research is not only to gather good data but to develop a society in which all people are healthy and are empowered to remain that way.

Notes

1. Research in progress uses a pretest-posttest quasi-experimental design, with the video serving as the treatment. Short surveys test hantavirus knowledge before exposure to the video

and other educational materials. The survey referred to here was a pilot study conducted at local health fairs. This research will continue with a more appropriate (to the population) 7-minute video that is in production at the time of this writing.

2. Like spoken English, which differs from region to region throughout the United States, spoken Spanish differs from country to country and region to region. These differences also reflect differences in social class, educational background, and subcultural identification. In other words, migrant and seasonal farmworkers have a dialect distinct to their regional origins and to their cultural group. Further, it is commonly held that "border Spanish" is a unique dialect that blends Mexican Spanish and southwestern American English, along with an argot or slang specific to the border region. Although the migrants could certainly understand standard and proper Spanish (of which Castillian is an exemplar), it is not *their* language per se. See Mody (1991) and Windahl and Signitzer (1992) for developmental communication message design strategies.

References

Bremner, J. A. (1993). Hantavirus infections and outbreaks in 1993. *CDR Review, 4,* R5-R9.

Brown, L., & Tandon, R. (1983). Ideology and political economy in inquiry: Action research and participatory research. *Journal of Applied and Behavioral Science, 19,* 277-294.

Centers for Disease Control and Prevention. (1994). *Preventing hantavirus disease* [Video]. Atlanta: Author.

Foster, C. (1996, May 21). Columbus trustees put community health clinic on hold. *Las Cruces Sun-News,* p. 4.

Geist, P. (1994). Negotiating cultural understanding in health care communication. In L. Samovar & R. Porter (Eds.), *Intercultural communication* (pp. 311-321). Belmont, CA: Wadsworth.

Hall, B. (1981). Participatory research, popular knowledge and power. *Convergence, 14*(3), 6-17.

Howe-Murphy, R., Ross, G., Tseng, R., & Hartwig, R. (1989). Effecting change in multicultural health promotion: A systems approach. *Journal of Allied Health, 18,* 291-305.

Jones, S. (1982). Social marketing: Dimensions of power and politics. *European Journal of Marketing, 16,* 46-53.

Kaplan, D., Alpert, J., Blodgett, F., & Gargas, D. (1989). Health care for children of migrant families. *Pediatrics, 84,* 739-740.

Korzenny, F., & Ting-Toomey, S. (Eds.). (1992). *Mass media effects across cultures.* Newbury Park, CA: Sage.

Kreeger, K. Y. (1994, July 25). One year later, the hantavirus investigation continues. *Scientist,* pp. 15, 17.

Lefebvre, R. C., Doner, L., Johnston, C., Loughrey, K., Balch, G. I., & Sutton, S. M. (1995). Use of database marketing and consumer-based health communication in message design: An example from the Office of Cancer Communications' "5 a Day for Better Health" program. In E. Maibach & R. L. Parrott (Eds.), *Designing health messages: Approaches from communication theory and public health practice* (pp. 217-246). Thousand Oaks, CA: Sage.

Lemonick, M. (1993, December 6). Closing in on a mysterious killer. *Time,* pp. 66-67.

Manning, A. (1996, June 12). Global team to track disease. *USA Today,* p. 1.

Mody, B. (1991). *Designing messages for development communication: An audience participation-based approach.* Newbury Park, CA: Sage.

Nair, K. S., & White, S. A. (1993). *Perspectives on development communication.* Newbury Park, CA: Sage.

Ratzan, S. C., Payne, J. G., & Massett, H. A. (1994). Effective health message design: The America Responds to AIDS campaign. *American Behavioral Scientist, 38,* 294-309.

Ray, E. B. (Ed.). (1996). *Communication and disenfranchisement: Social health issues and implications.* Mahwah, NJ: Lawrence Erlbaum.

Reckitt & Coleman, Inc. (1994a). *Answers to frequently asked questions about hantavirus* [Pamphlet]. (Available from their hantavirus helpline, 1-800-395-3266)

Reckitt & Coleman, Inc. (1994b). *Hantavirus: The essential facts* [Pamphlet]. (Available from their hantavirus helpline, 1-800-395-3266)

Reckitt & Coleman, Inc. (1995). *Hantavirus: Information about the disease and how to help prevent it* [Pamphlet]. (Available from their hantavirus helpline, 1-800-395-3266)

Rogers, E. (1995). *Diffusion of innovations* (4th ed.). New York: Free Press.

Sands, L., Kioski, C., & Komatus, K. (1993). Hantavirus in the southwestern U.S.: Epidemiology of an emerging pathogen. *Journal of the American Osteopathic Association, 93,* 1279-1285.

Severin, W., & Tankard, J. (1992). *Communication theories: Origins, methods and uses in the mass media.* New York: Longman.

Tandon, R. (1981). Participatory research in the empowerment of people. *Convergence, 14*(3), 20-29.

Van Maanen, J. (1988). *Tales of the field.* Chicago: University of Chicago Press.

Wenzel, R. (1994). A new hantavirus infection in North America. *New England Journal of Medicine, 330,* 1004-1005.

Wieder, D. L., & Hartsell, H. (1996, May). *Community as a folk concept in public health planning.* Paper presented at the annual meeting of the International Communication Association, Chicago.

Windahl, S., & Signitzer, B. (1992). *Using communication theory.* Newbury Park, CA: Sage.

Witte, K. (1995). Fishing for success: Using the persuasive health message framework for generating effective campaign messages. In E. Maibach & R. L. Parrott (Eds.), *Designing health messages: Approaches from communication theory and public health practice* (pp. 145-166). Thousand Oaks, CA: Sage.

Part 2

∽∾

Challenges of Two
Adjoining Health Systems

Proximity has long been a topic of research for social scientists. Psychologists and social psychologists have been interested in understanding the influence of affiliation and association, going back to the pioneering work of Georg Simmel. Sociologists and anthropologists have also been interested in proximity in terms of demographic shifts among groups as well as the network patterns of group members. Public health researchers are particularly interested in proximity and personal contact to understand the spread of epidemics. In general, all of these interested parties share one focus: How does the proximity of one agent influence the attitudes and behavior of the other?

The case of the proximity of the United States and Mexico is particularly interesting because the two environments are so radically different. The United States is regarded as a first-world industrialized country that has a predominantly Protestant culture and that treats English as the official language. Mexico, on the other hand, has a less developed economy that is rurally based, it is predominantly Catholic, and Spanish is the official language. Because of the difference in the economies, the resources available for health services are much greater in the United States than in Mexico but proportionately less in U.S. border regions than in the rest of the United States. The difference in religious values influences perceptions of responsibility and views regarding morality. Language differences also create obstacles in the delivery and comprehension of health messages, particularly when English-language materials are used with Spanish-speaking populations, as is much more common than the reverse.

The four articles in this section address how the unique proximity of the United States and Mexico influences the attitudes and health-related behaviors of the population living in the border region. An underlying assumption of the four chapters is that the legal border that separates the two countries is somewhat porous and that the interaction between the people from both regions gives rise to the unique hybrid environment that is the borderlands of the United States and Mexico. This hybridization is manifested in the range of mass media messages disseminated, the variety of health services available, the different sexual practices prevailing in both regions, and the contrasting laws guiding availability of medications.

Chapter 5

∽∾

ALCOHOL AND TOBACCO ADVERTISING IN THE BORDER REGION

J. GERARD POWER

"Getting people to change their private behavior, for the public good, or even for their own well-being, has been a chronic national problem."

Jesse Green, "Flirting With Suicide,"
New York Times Magazine (September 15, 1996, p. 40)

The quotation above was written in reference to the increasing numbers engaging in unsafe sexual practices despite a decade of public health campaigns designed to persuade people to protect themselves when having sex. This general sentiment reflects the burgeoning criticism of health campaign attempts by agencies and organizations to influence a host of health-related behaviors, including safe sex practices, teen pregnancy, and alcohol and tobacco consumption. At the same time, public health researchers and practitioners are increasingly concerned about the influence of media and advertising on sexual behavior, drinking, and smoking (Atkin, Hocking, & Block, 1984; Harms & Wolk, 1990). One explanation for these two inconsistent outcomes is that commercial advertisers have managed to integrate more persuasive strategies into their messages than their counterparts in public health.

This explanation opens up an avenue of investigation that brings together the literatures on health promotion and mass communication

(Atkin & Wallack, 1990; Backer, Rogers, & Sopory, 1992; Gilman, 1995; Kreps & Kunimoto, 1994; Maibach & Parrott, 1995). Persuasive messages, whether they are commercial advertisements for tobacco and alcohol products or public service announcements advocating smoking cessation or moderation in alcohol consumption, may succeed or fail for the same or similar reasons. The key to the success of tobacco and alcohol advertising and the explanation for the lack of success of public health campaigns may lie in how these messages are affected by contextual aspects of people's lives, including language(s) spoken, ethnic identity, and geographic location of the target audience (Schudson, 1984; Witte & Morrison, 1995).

These issues are of particular interest to the border region of the southwestern United States, which is home to a largely poor, Hispanic, and Spanish-speaking population. This population is characterized by high unemployment and low literacy levels, but federal and state resources are disproportionately distributed to other parts of the four respective border states (Suárez y Toriello & Chávez, 1996). That these characteristics are related to the public health of this population is a viewpoint that is gaining increasing support. For example, Williams, Lavizzo-Mourey, and Warren (1994) highlighted the variety of ways in which health status in the United States is tied to race and ethnicity.

There are three main reasons that the border region provides useful illustrations of the relationship between advertising and health behavior. First, as the numbers and spending power of Hispanics have increased, so also has the amount of alcohol and tobacco advertising targeted at this market (Maxwell & Jacobson, 1989). Second, prior research has confirmed that poor ethnic communities are exposed to more alcohol and tobacco advertising than their wealthier Anglo counterparts (Hackbarth, Silvestri, & Cosper, 1995). Third, in the United States, the Federal Communications Commission regulates the advertising of tobacco and alcohol on U.S. television (Schuster & Pacelli Powell, 1987). However, television channels originating in Mexico are not subject to such extreme restrictions (A. N. Barrios, personal communication, July 1996; A. F. Navarro, personal communication, July 1996). The combination of these factors presents a unique set of circumstances for Spanish-speaking television viewers in the border region. Because of the proximity to Mexico, border populations receive both U.S. TV channels and Spanish-language TV from Mexico. To the extent that advertising is effective, one would expect higher consumption of alcohol and cigarettes among Spanish-speaking Mexican Americans living in border communities than among Mexican Americans living in other parts of the country. This example of cross-border media influence will be discussed, and the available data on alcohol consumption and cigarette smoking among Mexican Americans on the border will be examined. The findings will be analyzed in the context of the need for binational regulation on advertising in general and television advertising in particular in border communities.

This chapter examines the theory and research on tobacco and alcohol advertising, focusing on three interrelated themes: (a) the research evidence on the effects of advertising on smoking and drinking patterns in general; (b) the growing literature on how advertising disproportionately targets certain groups within specific geographic locations, particularly the Hispanic population; and (c) the relationship between culture and advertising and how such contextual aspects as language, ethnicity, and immigrant status influence receptivity to persuasive messages. These three themes provide the basis for a discussion of the role of tobacco and alcohol advertising in the border region that separates and joins the United States and Mexico. Finally, a research agenda is proposed to further explore the phenomenon of alcohol and tobacco advertising to Hispanics in the border region.

Advertising Alcohol and Tobacco

Theoretical explanations abound on the relationship between advertising and alcohol consumption (Harms & Wolk, 1990). The effects of advertising on drinking and smoking behavior are predicated on the ubiquity, frequency, salience, and cumulative nature of messages advocating alcohol and tobacco use in one's personal environment (Blum, 1991; Krupka, Vener, & Richmond, 1990). For example, Madden and Grube (1994) examined the frequency and nature of alcohol and tobacco advertising in a random sample of 166 televised sports events representing 443.7 hours of network programming broadcast from the fall of 1990 through the summer of 1992. The authors reported that there were more commercials for alcohol products than for any other beverage and that beer commercials were predominant. Further, multiple exposure to product names and labels was achieved through stadium signs, on-site promotions, and verbal and visual brief product sponsorships.

Building on a differential association hypothesis, Harms and Wolk (1990) argued that "drinking occurs when positive perceptions of drinking outweigh or outnumber negative ones" (p. 21). Advertising of alcohol and tobacco is clearly centered on the association of these drugs with positive perceptions. Further, the positive consequences of this association are likely to influence the extent to which certain behaviors are modeled. The implications of this association, however, are somewhat more difficult to prove. Atkin et al. (1984) noted the favorable portrayals of drinkers in alcohol ads as youthful, happy, physically attractive, and successful. Further, these attributes correspond accurately with and are likely to facilitate many of the reasons young people give for drinking, including social acceptance, conformity, and escape. The authors reported that in a study of 665 teenagers from the 7th through 12th grades in Michigan, California, New York, and Georgia, "Peer influence is clearly the strongest correlate of beer drinking, followed by exposure to beer advertising" (p. 162). The authors also demonstrated a positive correlation between exposure to liquor advertising and liquor drinking.

A similar study of 602 junior high school students from Grades 7 and 8 by Botvin, Goldberg, Botvin, and Dusenbury (1993) examined the relationship between smoking prevalence and exposure to cigarette advertisements. The findings suggested that exposure to cigarette advertising and having friends who smoked were the strongest predictors of current smoking status. Consequently, adolescents with high exposure to cigarette advertising were significantly more likely to be smokers than were those with low exposure to cigarette advertising.

In a review of the debate between the tobacco and alcohol industry and public health advocates, Orlandi, Lieberman, and Schinke (1989) examined the evidence of the relationship between advertising exposure and smoking and drinking behavior (see also Tye, Warner, & Glantz, 1987). Rejecting the validity of a direct effects relationship, Orlandi et al. (1989) proposed examining the factors that are known to be predictors of substance abuse and the ways in which ads are most likely to influence them. In the case of adolescents, for example, family and peer influences as well as the formation of personal identity have been demonstrated to be strongly correlated with tobacco and alcohol use. These factors then serve as the contextual variables that frame the promotion of tobacco and alcohol products.

One of the greatest challenges to counteracting the effects of alcohol and tobacco advertising is the relationship between the alcohol and tobacco industry and commercial mass media systems, particularly in the United States and increasingly in other parts of the world. For example, Weis and Burke (1986) documented evidence to support the belief that commercial media in the United States have avoided addressing the health risks caused by smoking because of the fear of losing large advertising revenue. This evidence includes the deletion of text adverse to smoking by the weekly newsmagazines *Newsweek* and *Time* in advertising supplements written to educate readers on the basics of personal health care. Even though the promotion of tobacco products is banned, television also engages in self-censorship because the networks receive millions of dollars to advertise many nontobacco products manufactured by companies owned entirely or in part by Philip Morris and R. J. Reynolds, the large tobacco companies.

The comparison, therefore, between tobacco and alcohol advertising and health promotion campaigns to reduce cigarette and alcohol consumption is not a fair one. In a review of alcohol advertising and health promotion efforts, Harms and Wolk (1990) juxtaposed what they termed "agencies of promotion" and "agencies of prevention." They argued that there are major differences in the organization and resources of these two agencies. First, because alcoholic beverage companies regard advertising as a central component of their business enterprise, there is a regular budget allocation for promotional activities, including advertising. These resources are not always available to health agencies and organizations. Second, national communication campaigns for alcohol advertising are usually planned and implemented by advertising agency experts. Health agencies and organizations usually do not have the expertise or resources to plan such sophisticated and complex media campaigns. Third, advertising is a tax-deductible expense, so the cost of alcohol advertising is actually subsidized indirectly by taxpayers and the public. Although this use of tax money is very discreet, the public is much more aware that it is supporting health campaign efforts, and consequently public health agencies and organizations are subject to greater public scrutiny and criticism. In terms of public health services and commercial advertising strategies, Hispanics in the U.S.-Mexico border region serve as an interesting case study.

Targeting Hispanics: Ethnicity and Geography

Research over the last 10 years in particular has documented the disproportionate lack of access and availability of health care services to Hispanics relative to other ethnic groups in the United States. In some cases, the geographic location and distribution of Hispanics have been argued to contribute to the low level of health services. At the same time, ethnicity and geographic location have also served as strategic parameters for advertising and marketing alcohol and tobacco to Hispanics. This section juxta-poses these two patterns and identifies the criteria used to promote alcohol and tobacco consumption among Hispanics.

In the United States, Hispanics constitute a seriously underserved population with regard to health care services. Valdez, Giachello, Rodriguez-Trias, Gomez, and De la Rocha (1993) reported that in California and Texas, Hispanics account for a major share of the uninsured population. In the last 10 years, the number of uninsured Hispanics increased by 151%, composed mainly of communities of Mexican and Central American origin. Aguirre-Molina, Ramirez, and Ramirez (1993) reported that compared with other groups in the United States, Hispanics are least likely to have medical care benefits such as health insurance, Medicaid, and regular sources of care. In particular, Hispanic youth and older adults make fewer health care visits per year than do non-Hispanic whites. A study of 140 immigrant Mexican women in southern California reported that being discriminated against was the strongest of 12 measures of stress used in predicting high scores on a scale of depressive symptoms (Salgado de Snyder, 1987).

The relationship between health risk, access to resources, and geo-graphic location has received increasing attention from health researchers and practitioners. For example, Williams et al. (1994) suggested that the relatively low level of dental visits among Mexican Americans may be partly due to their high concentration in the Southwest region, "where coverage of human services programs is not particularly generous" (p. 32). In addition, there is also a strong association between alcohol consumption and the availability of alcohol. This availability is often facilitated by more lenient licensing laws controlling the retail outlets for the sale of alcohol in poor and ethnic neighborhoods as opposed to wealthier and "whiter" areas (Rabow & Watt, 1984). The specific concern about cross-border advertising of alcohol and tobacco in this study is consistent with prior research that identifies the disproportionate exposure to advertisements based on geographic and sociodemographic factors.

Advertising in general and tobacco and alcohol advertising in particu-lar have expanded dramatically on a global level. This expansion has serious health, economic, and cultural implications for underdeveloped countries (Wallack & Montgomery, 1992). The advertisements for alcohol and tobacco products systematically ignore the health risk associated with use of the product: "With products such as alcohol and tobacco, the benefits tend to be intangible (prestige, status) and irrelevant to the product. . . . Healthy and successful models in the ads convey the basic theme that product use will contribute to the wealth and success of the consumer" (p. 215). As in the countries of the developed world, the revenues from advertising are a primary support for many mass media systems in the developing world. Consequently, there is usually very little profit motive for media systems to provide health-related information to media consumers. The effect of commercial forces in less developed countries is illustrated in a study comparing television and textbook content in Mexico, where children demonstrated a higher awareness of advertising images, symbols, and slogans than of the images and symbols associated with the nation's history (Murdock & Janus, 1984).

On a more local level, recent research has confirmed the belief that certain geographic areas are more heavily saturated with alcohol and tobacco advertising. Hackbarth et al. (1995) conducted a cross-sectional prevalence survey of all billboards located within the city of Chicago. The researchers compared the combined number of alcohol and tobacco billboards in white versus minority wards and found a mean of 20 billboards in white wards versus a mean of 74 alcohol and tobacco billboards in minority wards. In other words, "A child walking to school in an African-American or Hispanic neighborhood is three times more likely to see a tobacco billboard than a child residing in a predominantly white neighborhood" (p. 224).

Finally, in addition to the predatory advertising practices of the alcohol and tobacco industry, illegal sales of alcohol and tobacco are also more likely to occur in low-income, inner-city communities with high concentrations of ethnic minorities. These are also the areas where there are high concentrations of alcohol outlets and high rates of alcohol-related youth violence (Mosher, 1995; Mosher & Works, 1994; Preusser & Williams, 1992). Clearly, geographic segmentation serves to disproportionately target alcohol and tobacco promotional messages as well as availability of these products to ethnic minorities.

The increasing size and spending power of the Hispanic market have led advertisers to pay more attention and to target their promotional materials more strategically to Hispanics than ever before. Maxwell and Jacobson (1989) stated that "the Hispanic market is the hottest one around, . . . and beer, cigarette, and junk food producers are going after it in a big way. Unfortunately, those products promote drunk driving, cancer, heart disease and obesity—diseases that are widespread or growing rapidly in the Hispanic community" (back cover).

The tobacco industry spends almost $4 billion per year advertising cigarette smoking (Hackbarth et al., 1995). Alcohol is linked with 100,000 deaths per year, and cigarettes are linked with more than 350,000 (Kilbourne, 1991; Mosher, 1995).

In the United States, Hispanics are reported to have some of the highest rates of consumption of alcoholic beverages. Usage rates for nicotine also indicate that Hispanics generally smoke more than non-Hispanic whites. Further, Mexican Americans between the ages of 35 and 74 smoke more than any other Hispanic ethnic group (Marín, Posner, & Kinyon, 1993). Gilbert and Cervantes (1986) reported that both Mexican men and Mexican women drink more during each drinking episode than other male and female drinkers in the United States.

Alcohol and tobacco advertising has also been designed specifically for the Hispanic market. Taylor (1990) identified a range of tobacco and alcohol advertising campaigns that are targeted directly at Hispanics. The author also noted the growing concern about the escalating cancer rates among Hispanics and the fact that more Hispanics are smoking and are smoking more cigarettes than in the past. In addition, alcohol-related problems, which had been limited almost exclusively to men, are now spreading to Hispanic women, who traditionally drank little. This concern was echoed by Hackbarth et al. (1995), who noted the focus on Hispanics, particularly Hispanic women, in advertising campaigns by Newport, Winston, Camel, Salem, Rio, Dorado, and other brands. Tye et al. (1987) noted that cigarette advertising, which is now extremely common in magazines such as *Hispanic Times* and *Hispano Americano,* barely existed before 1984. "Brands such as Rio and Dorado are targeted at Hispanics, making Philip Morris the single biggest advertiser in Hispanic media, with R. J. Reynolds not far behind" (Pollay, Lee, & Carter-Whitney, 1995, p. 111; see also Fitch, 1986; Levin, 1988). The Office of Minority Health reported in 1985 that smoking rates among Mexican American youths far exceeded those of their non-Hispanic white and African American counterparts (Tye et al., 1987).

For Mexican Americans, the proximity to Mexico also reinforces Mexican rather than American drinking and smoking patterns and makes it more difficult for recent arrivals to adapt to the cultural mores of the host culture (Hurtado, 1995). In a similar vein, Dusenbury, Epstein, Botvin, and Diaz (1994) examined the relationship between language spoken and smoking among 3,129 Hispanic students in 47 New York City public and parochial schools. The findings indicate that being bicultural (speaking both English and Spanish) at home and with friends appeared to increase the odds of currently smoking (for boys but not girls). One interpretation of this finding offered by the authors is that smoking may alleviate some of the tension and stress associated with biculturalism (see also Fitzpatrick, 1987).

Noting the importance of language fluency, Marín (1994) conducted two studies with 1,204 Hispanics (Study 1) and 1,569 Hispanics (Study 2) to establish their level of awareness of product warning messages and signs. The author reported that less acculturated Spanish-speaking Hispanics are less likely to report being aware of the product warning messages (e.g., for alcoholic beverages), particularly those that appear only in English. A similar concern about the uselessness of warning labels was voiced by Snyder and Blood (1992), who provided evidence that these messages may actually be counterproductive. The authors conducted an experiment to test the effects of the newly introduced Surgeon General's alcohol warnings and advertisements on college students. The findings suggest that the warning labels are overpowered by the images and messages in the advertisement. Consequently, the warnings may serve to legitimize the product by implying that despite the risk involved, multiple benefits can be accrued by consumption of the product.

The research evidence, therefore, suggests that advertisers promoting alcohol and cigarettes have been much more successful than public health researchers and practitioners at influencing their consumers. In addition to the structural and organizational differences between agencies of promotion and prevention (Harms & Wolk, 1990), the fundamental difference in the two strategies is based on a more focused attention to the relationship between culture and promotional messages.

Culture and Promotional Messages

This section draws on a range of literatures that attempt to understand the relationship between culture and promotional messages. The discussion focuses specifically on Hispanics in the border region and the differential impacts of advertising versus health promotional messages. Harms and Wolk (1990) identified a range of relevant characteristics of alcohol advertising. First, there is a direct association between the product and a range of emotional cognitive faculties, in the tradition of classical conditioning. Alaniz and Wilkes (1995) suggested that alcohol advertising to Mexican Americans "offers the promise of a new world of urban comfort, female companionship and assuredness" (p. 436). Second, certain symbols, such as places and people, are selected to evoke a particular response in the audience. Many beer advertisements to Mexican Americans contain "familiar components of Mexican culture . . . tiled bars and staircases, maps on swimsuits, authentic furniture and architecture" (Alaniz & Wilkes, 1995, p. 436). Third, very little product information is communicated to consumers. To the extent that this might be understandable to a monolingual Spanish consumer, the information is not available. Even government health warnings are not effective, either because they are not understood or because they are overpowered by the visual components of the rest of the ad and consequently ignored. Fourth, alcohol and tobacco advertising must be examined in the aggregate and in terms of its cumulative effects rather than in isolated individual alcohol or tobacco advertising messages.

The complexity of alcohol and tobacco advertising appeals requires an approach that is not reductionist. Consequently, the failure of social scientists to demonstrate conclusively that viewing tobacco or alcohol ads has a direct causal effect on the use of these products does not refute the argument that advertising is extremely effective in influencing behavior (Orlandi et al., 1989). The complexity of the relationship between advertising and culture is expressed by Alaniz and Wilkes (1995), who suggested that

> by drawing on the images of the lifeworld employed among Hispanic groups, commodity producers attempt to control the principal domains of cultural value in order to increase their brand's currency in the market and to control consumption and high market share. Thus, in the case of the alcohol industry and the Mexican American community, advertising seeks to draw on images of Mexican mythology, history, tradition, culture, and language to more adequately secure a foothold in the commodity process. (p. 433)

Thus, images in alcohol and cigarette advertisements serve as "social experiences" (Harms & Wolk, 1990) on which cultural assumptions about drinking and smoking are based. They become cultural referents or benchmarks that establish the norms for what is perceived as appropriate and acceptable. These benchmarks facilitate one's understanding of what it is to be cool and accepted by one's peers; to be male or macho, female or feminine; to be Mexican; and to have status (see Alaniz & Wilkes, 1995, for a semiotic analysis of a range of alcohol advertisements targeted at the Mexican American community).

Advertising to Hispanics in the Borderlands

In Hispanic communities throughout the border region of the United States and Mexico, one is bombarded with gigantic billboards of the Marlboro man, the Virginia Slims girl, Joe Camel, and Kool cigarettes. Neighborhood grocery stores, auto mechanic shops, and taco stands are full of the icons of alcohol and tobacco advertising displayed on posters, calendars, and neon signs. These include the images of masculinity—the bullfighter, the mariachi, and the charro—and of bikini-clad, (usually) blonde models, often with beer brands and the stereotypic symbols of Mexican nationalism (the flag, the map of Mexico, and Aztec iconography) depicted on their swimsuits.

Of alcohol advertising in the Mexican American community, Alaniz and Wilkes (1995) suggested that

> the sign system of Mexican-American communities is encoded from the outside to reflect the needs of alcohol markets, while the authentic images of human lives are lost and distorted. These distortions play themselves out in the most concrete of social pathologies, in particular, in widespread patterns of alcohol abuse and related community problems. (p. 445)

This relationship between alcohol consumption and social problems in the Mexican American population is demonstrated in a study by Caetano and Medina-Mora (1988) comparing drinking patterns among Mexican Americans and Mexican nationals. Maxwell and Jacobson (1989) have also connected the rise in health problems related to food, tobacco, and advertising with the huge increase in the level of Hispanic-specific advertising.

Located in the southwestern United States, El Paso, Texas, is the largest city on the U.S.-Mexico border. Nearly three quarters (73.5%) of its population is Hispanic (Texas Department of Health, 1995). Most of this population is Spanish speaking. El Paso and the border region have the second highest level of acute alcohol risk in the state of Texas (Texas Department of Health, 1995). In a survey of high school students sponsored by the *El Paso Times* and KVIA-Channel 7, more than two in three seniors (68%) reported drinking in the past 30 days (Moore, 1996). This rate is far above the national average reported in other studies. In the 1994 Texas Youth Behavior Risk Study, 20.2% of students in Grade 6 reported using tobacco in the last school year, and 37.9% of the same group reported consuming alcohol during the same period. A comparison of tobacco consumption by ethnic group indicates that tobacco is used by 18.5% of non-Hispanic whites and 21.1% of Mexican Americans. The difference between these two groups is far greater for alcohol use, with 29.1% of non-Hispanic whites reporting alcohol use in comparison with 40.0% of Mexican Americans.

Physical proximity to Ciudad Juárez and its more lenient drinking laws and less expensive alcohol and cigarettes may be contributing factors to the differences between Mexican Americans and non-Hispanic whites (see Chapter 3 of this book). Another part of the puzzle is that the Spanish-speaking population may be exposed to disproportionate amounts of alcohol and cigarette advertising in the United States and on television channels originating in Mexico. Television is the preferred medium for obtaining news and information. According to the *Gallup Poll Monthly* (Moore, 1995), 78% of Americans get their news regularly from television. In El Paso, the stations broadcasting from Mexico are XHJCI and XHJUB (Televisa), XHCH and XEPM (Television Azteca), XHIJ (Telemundo), and XEJ (Univision).

Interviews with representatives of Mexican television stations in Ciudad Juárez indicate that alcoholic beverages can be advertised after 10:00 p.m. and cigarettes after 9:00 p.m. (A. N. Barrios, personal communication, July 1996; A. F. Navarro, personal communication, July 1996). Because of the 1-hour time difference between El Paso and Ciudad Juárez, alcohol advertising is broadcast from Mexican television stations after 9:00 p.m. in El Paso and cigarette advertising after 8:00 p.m. However, it is important to note that lobbyists in Mexico are fighting to further restrict the amount and frequency of alcohol and tobacco advertising available on Mexican television (A. F. Navarro, personal communication, July 1996).

A Research Agenda

The literature reviewed in this chapter points to the value of a number of interrelated lines of research. It would be valuable (a) to identify the contextual variables—language, social class/status, ethnicity—associated with Hispanics living in border regions; (b) to establish the extent to which these contextual variables are associated with the appeal of cigarette smoking and alcohol consumption; (c) to conduct a content analysis to examine the prevalence of these appeals in alcohol and tobacco advertisements on both sides of the U.S.-Mexico border; and (d) to explore the potential to integrate counterappeals that draw on the same contextual variables in public health campaigns to reduce smoking and alcohol consumption.

Conclusions

The purpose of this chapter was to integrate a range of literatures to explain the differential effects of public health campaigns and commercial advertising on alcohol and tobacco consumption in the Hispanic community, with a special focus on the U.S.-Mexico border region. First, we reviewed research on the relationship between advertising and alcohol and tobacco consumption that highlighted the difficulty of establishing such effects. Second, we examined the research connecting the relatively recent targeting of Hispanics by alcoholic beverage and tobacco companies to a rise in health problems associated with these behaviors. Of particular note was the research on how poor ethnic neighborhoods have been especially bombarded with advertisements for alcohol and tobacco products. Third, we examined the relationship between culture and advertising in an attempt to partly explain why advertising appears to work when health campaigns do not.

Hispanics living in the border region of the United States and Mexico were cited as an example of a population that has relatively high levels of alcohol consumption and cigarette smoking. What is unique about this particular population is that it is exposed not only to multiple advertisements in the United States but also, because of its proximity to Mexico, to both alcohol and cigarette advertising on multiple TV channels originating in Mexico. This situation raises all of the classic arguments that have been waged against the alcoholic beverage and tobacco industries in the United States, with the added complexity of the cumulative effects of alcohol and cigarette commercials that are being beamed unobstructed from Mexico. To the extent that legislators can be convinced of the complex nature of the relationship between advertising and its effects, this situation demands some form of binational regulation of alcohol and cigarette advertising on Mexican TV channels available in the United States.

Finally, what lessons can public health campaigns designed to reduce alcohol use and smoking among Hispanics learn from commercial advertisements created to promote drinking and smoking in the same population? First, there is a clear pattern in associating the consumption of the product with favorable emotions, such as happiness, satisfaction, love, and security.

This is in stark contrast to the emphasis on negative messages and fear appeals in many public health campaigns. Second, commercial advertisements for alcohol and tobacco appeal to the need for peer approval, to be included, to be able to conform. Many public health campaigns focus on encouraging one to stand apart from the crowd—a difficult task for those learning how to adapt to a new culture. Third, alcohol and tobacco ads contain multiple images and symbols that are easily identifiable to the target audience, often appealing to cultural stereotypes and notions of ethnic and national identity. Again, this contrasts with the anonymous figure/character that often appears in public health campaigns targeting specific behaviors. Finally, studies designed to evaluate the effects of health campaigns cannot rely on reductionist models of cause-and-effect relationships—in this case, how exposure directly affects alcohol and cigarette consumption.

In conclusion, this chapter has attempted to address the vulnerability of Hispanics in the border region to alcohol and tobacco advertisements. It constitutes a first step in identifying the contributing factors to the high rates of alcohol consumption and cigarette smoking in this population. Through this analysis it has also attempted to highlight the differences between commercial advertising campaigns and public health campaigns. The unique issue of cross-border advertising highlighted in this chapter warrants further research attention to substantiate the degree to which these ads originating in Mexico affect their U.S. consumers. This is one more challenge to a cross-border health initiative.

References

Aguirre-Molina, M., Ramirez, A., & Ramirez, M. (1993). Health promotion and disease prevention strategies. *Public Health Reports, 108,* 559-564.

Alaniz, M. L., & Wilkes, C. (1995). Reinterpreting Latino culture in the commodity form: The case of alcohol advertising in the Mexican American community. *Hispanic Journal of Behavioral Sciences, 17,* 430-451.

Atkin, C., Hocking, J., & Block, M. (1984). Teenage drinking: Does advertising make a difference? *Journal of Communication, 34,* 157-167.

Atkin, C., & Wallack, L. (1990). *Mass communication and public health: Complexities and conflicts.* Thousand Oaks, CA: Sage.

Backer, T. E., Rogers, E. M., & Sopory, P. (1992). *Designing health communication campaigns: What works?* Newbury Park, CA: Sage.

Blum, A. (1991). The Marlboro Grand Prix: Circumvention of the television ban on tobacco advertising. *New England Journal of Medicine, 324,* 913-917.

Botvin, G. J., Goldberg, C. J., Botvin, E. M., & Dusenbury, L. (1993). Smoking behavior of adolescents exposed to cigarette advertising. *Public Health Reports, 108,* 217-224.

Caetano, R., & Medina Mora, M. E. (1988). Patrones de consumo de alcohol y problemas asociados en Mexico y en población de origen Mexicano que habita en Estados Unidos. *Nueva Antropología, 10,* 137-155.

Dusenbury, L., Epstein, J. A., Botvin, G. J., & Diaz, T. (1994). The relationship between language spoken and smoking among Hispanic-Latino youth in New York City. *Public Health Reports, 109,* 421-427.

Fitch, E. (1986, February 27). Hispanic marketing: Prime space available at low rates. *Advertising Age,* p. 11.

Fitzpatrick, J. P. (1987). *Puerto Rican Americans: The meaning of migration to the mainland.* Englewood Cliffs, NJ: Prentice Hall.

Gilbert, J. M., & Cervantes, R. C. (1986). Patterns and practices of alcohol use among Mexican Americans: A comprehensive review. *Hispanic Journal of Behavioral Sciences, 8,* 1-53.

Gilman, S. L. (1995). *Picturing health and illness: Images of identity and difference.* Baltimore: Johns Hopkins University Press.

Green, J. (1996, September 15). Flirting with suicide. *New York Times Magazine,* p. 39.

Hackbarth, D. P., Silvestri, B., & Cosper, W. (1995). Tobacco and alcohol billboards in 50 Chicago neighborhoods: Market segmentation to sell dangerous products to the poor. *Journal of Public Health Policy, 16,* 213-230.

Harms, J. B., & Wolk, J. L. (1990). Differential perception and adolescent drinking in the United States: Preliminary considerations. *Journal of Sociology and Social Welfare, 49,* 21-41.

Hurtado, R. (1995). *Where saying no is not enough.* Unpublished manuscript, Department of Communication, University of Texas at El Paso.

Kilbourne, J. (1991). Deadly persuasion: The case against advertising of "legal" drugs. *Propaganda Review, 9,* 29-33.

Kreps, G. L., & Kunimoto, N. (1994). *Effective communication in multicultural health settings.* Thousand Oaks, CA: Sage.

Krupka, L. R., Vener, A. M., & Richmond, G. (1990). Tobacco advertising in gender-oriented popular magazines. *Journal of Drug Education, 21,* 15-29.

Levin, M. (1988). The tobacco industry's strange bedfellows. *Business and Society Review, 65,* 11-17.

Madden, P. A., & Grube, J. W. (1994). The frequency and nature of alcohol and tobacco advertising in televised sports, 1990 through 1992. *American Journal of Public Health, 84,* 297-299.

Maibach, E., & Parrott, R. (1995). *Designing health messages: Approaches from communication theory and public health practice.* Thousand Oaks, CA: Sage.

Marín, G. (1994). Self-reported awareness of the presence of product warning messages and signs by Hispanics in San Francisco. *Public Health Reports, 109,* 275-283.

Marín, G., Posner, S. F., & Kinyon, J. B. (1993). Alcohol expectancies among Hispanics and non-Hispanic whites: Role of drinking status and acculturation. *Hispanic Journal of Behavioral Sciences, 15,* 373-381.

Maxwell, B., & Jacobson, M. (1989). *Marketing disease to Hispanics.* Washington, DC: Center for Science in the Public Interest.

Moore, D. (1995, September). America's most important source of information: Local TV news. *Gallup Poll Monthly,* pp. 2-8.

Moore, R. (1996). *Class of '96 executive summary.* El Paso, TX: El Paso Times.

Mosher, J. F. (1995). The merchants, not the customers: Resisting the alcohol and tobacco industries' strategy to blame young people for illegal alcohol and tobacco sales. *Journal of Public Health Policy, 16,* 412-432.

Mosher, J. F., & Works, R. (1994). *Confronting Sacramento: State preemption, community, control, and alcohol outlet blight in two inner-city communities.* San Rafael, CA: Marin Institute for the Prevention of Alcohol and Other Drug Problems.

Murdock, G., & Janus, N. (1984). *Mass communication and the advertising industry* (Reports and Papers on Mass Communication No. 97). Paris: UNESCO.

Orlandi, M. A., Lieberman, L. R., & Schinke, S. P. (1989). The effects of alcohol and tobacco advertising on adolescents. *Perspectives on Adolescent Drug Use, 27,* 77-97.

Pollay, R. W., Lee, J. S., & Carter-Whitney, D. (1995). Separate but not equal: Racial segmentation in cigarette advertising. In G. Dines & J. M. Humez (Eds.), *Gender, race and class in media: A text-reader* (pp. 109-111). Thousand Oaks, CA: Sage.

Preusser, D., & Williams, A. (1992) Sales of alcohol to underage purchasers in three New York counties and Washington, D.C. *Journal of Public Health Policy, 13,* 306-317.

Rabow, J., & Watt, R. (1984). Alcohol availability, alcohol beverage sales and alcohol-related problems. *Journal for the Study of Alcohol, 43,* 747-801.

Salgado de Snyder, V. N. (1987). Factors associated with acculturative stress and depressive symptomatology among married Mexican immigrant women. *Psychological Women Quarterly, 11,* 475-488.

Schudson, M. (1984). *Advertising: The uneasy persuasion.* New York: Basic Books.

Schuster, C. P., & Pacelli Powell, C. (1987). Comparison of cigarette and alcohol advertising controversies. *Journal of Advertising, 16,* 26-33.

Snyder, L. B., & Blood, D. J. (1992, February). Caution: Alcohol advertising and the Surgeon General's alcohol warnings may have adverse effects on young adults. *Journal of Applied Communication Research,* pp. 37-53.

Suárez y Toriello, E., & Chavez, O. E. (1996). *Profile of the United States-Mexico border.* El Paso, TX: Federation of Private Associations for Community Development (FEMAP).

Taylor, P. (1990). Testimony on alcohol advertising: U.S. House of Representatives Subcommittee on Transportation and Hazardous Materials, March 1, 1990. *Journal of Public Health Policy, 11,* 370-381.

Texas Department of Health, Bureau of State Health Data and Policy Analysis. (1995). *Selected facts for El Paso County.* Austin: Author.

Tye, J. B., Warner, K. E., & Glantz, S. A. (1987). Tobacco advertising and consumption: Evidence of a causal relationship. *Journal of Public Health Policy, 8,* 492-508.

Valdez, R. B., Giachello, A., Rodriguez-Trias, H., Gomez, P., & De la Rocha, C. (1993). Improving access to health care in Latino communities. *Public Health Reports, 108,* 534-539.

Wallack, L., & Montgomery, K. (1992). Advertising for all by the year 2000: Public health implications for less developed countries. *Journal of Public Health Policy, 13,* 204-223.

Weis, W. L., & Burke, C. (1986). Media content and tobacco advertising: An unhealthy addiction. *Journal of Communication, 36,* 59-69.

Williams, D. R., Lavizzo-Mourey, R., & Warren, R. C. (1994). The concept of race and health status in America. *Public Health Reports, 109,* 26-41.

Witte, K., & Morrison, K. (1995). Intercultural and cross-cultural health communication: Understanding people and motivating health behaviors. In R. L. Wiseman (Ed.), *Intercultural communication theory* (pp. 216-246). Thousand Oaks, CA: Sage.

Chapter 6

∽∾

CROSS-BORDER COOPERATION

A Case Study of
Binational Tuberculosis Control

JILLIAN HOPEWELL

The U.S.-Mexico border region represents the physical and cultural interface between two large and different countries. The shared nature of this region presents a number of challenges for the administration and coordination of solutions for common concerns. In the case of health care, the presence of an artificial national boundary poses a number of difficulties, in particular for the control of infectious diseases. Many border communities are so closely linked that they must be considered as a single community in terms of the spread of infectious diseases, yet the presence of two separate public health systems often precludes a unified approach to disease control (Soberon, Valdez, & de Caso, 1989).

The United States and Mexico have periodically developed cooperative efforts to address specific public health concerns. Collaborative efforts between the United States and Mexico can prove complicated, given the political, administrative, and financial dynamics between these two countries. The purpose of this chapter is to examine two cases of local binational cooperation in tuberculosis control between the United States and Mexico. The two cases provide insight into issues of collaboration, the sustainability of binational programs, and barriers to success. As an outcome, this chapter will identify underlying design principles that facilitate the development and implementation of successful binational projects.

Mexican and U.S.
Public Health Systems

There are a number of differences between the public health systems of the United States and Mexico. These differences can create substantial difficulties and tension at the interface of the two systems along the U.S.-Mexico border. Mexico uses several parallel, highly centralized systems that have the advantage of consistency but lack flexibility and the ability to adapt to local circumstances. In the United States, public health care is more decentralized, leaving increased decision making at the local level but also creating a more disjointed overall health care system (Jacquart, 1994). To be effective, binational program designers and managers must take into account these fundamental differences and not expect either side to conform exactly to the other. It is largely for this reason that binational planners must not only understand the realities of each nation's public health system but be drawn from both nations.

Mexico's public health system is characterized by both fragmentation and centralization. Several different agencies are responsible for providing health care, but within each agency, all eyes turn toward Mexico City and, to a lesser extent, the state capitals, leaving few decision-making powers at the local level. Within the past decade, attempts have been made to change the health care system to one that is less centralized. To date, these attempts have been moderately successful in some areas, but the overall system remains (Gonzales-Block, 1993; Rodriguez, 1992).

The Mexican health care system is made up of three broad sectors: (a) social security, which includes the Instituto Mexicano de Seguro Social (Mexican Institute of Social Security [IMSS]) and the Instituto de Seguridad y Servicios Sociales para los Trabajadores del Estado (Institute of Security and Social Services for State Workers [ISSSTE]); (b) the Secretaria de Salud (Secretary of Health [SS]); and (c) the private sector.

The Mexican public health system began to emerge after the Mexican Revolution. During this time, the idea of health as a public good took hold. As a first step, the Cardenas administration (1934-1940) created the Secretaria de Asistencia Pública (Secretary of Public Assistance) and the Departamento de Salubridad (Department of Health). These two institutions were merged a few years later to become the Secretaria de Salud y Asistencia (Secretary of Health and Assistance). The Secretaria was charged with providing public health services to the poor and uninsured population. In 1943, Mexico created IMSS to meet the health care needs of Mexico's industrial workers and, soon after, its agricultural workers. In 1960, ISSSTE was created to serve government workers. Since the 1960s, several other smaller public health agencies have been established to serve very specific populations (Lopez Acuña, 1980). Examples include PEMEX, which serves Mexican oil workers, and IMSS-Solidaridad, designed to supply additional rural health care.

The private sector is a growing part of the health care system. Peter Ward (1986), in his book, *Welfare Politics in Mexico,* stated, "Nor is private medicine only a preserve of the rich. . . . The poor make extensive use of the private sector for 'lightweight' consultations, and they may also receive private treatment paid for by their employer" (p. 124). Though it is important not to discount the importance of the private health sector in Mexico, this study will focus on the public sector.

Table 6.1 shows the distribution of health care services among the major health agencies in Mexico in 1991.

The U.S. health care system is not nearly so centralized as that of Mexico, making the U.S. system more complex and difficult to sort out. The health care sector in the United States is made up of a variety of public, private, nonprofit, local, state, regional, and national organizations. Often these facilities cut across socioeconomic groups, making it more difficult to determine who goes where for care.

All federal government health policy comes under the aegis of the Department of Health and Human Services (DHHS), which was created in 1953. One of the primary responsibilities of the federal government is to develop and maintain data registries to track epidemiology trends in the nation. In addition, DHHS provides funding for many state- and local-level programs that cover a wide range of health care issues.

Within DHHS, the primary federal public health agency is the U.S. Public Health Service (USPHS), which was created by the U.S. Congress in 1912. Included within the USPHS are the Agency for Health Care Policy and Research, the Agency for Toxic Substances and Disease Registry, the Substance Abuse and Mental Health Services Administration, the Centers for Disease Control and Prevention (CDC), the Health Resources and

TABLE 6.1 Distribution of Health Care Services Among Major Health
Agencies in Mexico, 1991

Health Care Agency[a]	% of Outpatient Visits	% of Hospitalizations
SS	24.0	25.2
IMSS	53.6	53.0
ISSSTE	11.9	8.9
IMSS-Solidaridad	4.1	3.5
PEMEX	3.4	2.4
All others	3.0	7.0

SOURCE: Informe de Gobierno, Anexo, 1992, Mexico City, Mexico.
a. See text for definitions.

Services Administration (HRSA), the Indian Health Services, and the
National Institutes of Health (NIH). For the purposes of binational programs elaborated at the local level, the most important USPHS agencies
are HRSA and the CDC, with NIH also playing a significant role. It must
also be remembered that regional, state, and local public health entities will
have tremendous influence over binational health policy (General Accounting Office, 1988; Office of the Governor, 1993; Samuels, 1992).

The organizational differences between U.S. and Mexican public
health systems have enormous implications for the development of binational projects. One of the key differences between U.S. and Mexican
public health policy in the border region is that Mexico can make more
consistent policy decisions throughout the region because of agency centralization. It is easier for individual agencies in Mexico to show a united
front when implementing public health policy along the border or throughout the country. The disadvantage to this is that it leaves less room for
local-level innovations to keep pace with the realities in individual areas.

In both countries, the fact that health care delivery is dispersed among
a number of different entities means that it can be difficult to coordinate
programs. It may be somewhat simpler in the United States because the
state health departments are given clear responsibility for overseeing
reportable diseases (i.e., tuberculosis, human immunodeficiency virus
[HIV], sexually transmitted diseases, measles, and others) in most areas.
In both countries, effective disease prevention needs to include all of the
public health agencies in planning and implementation.

Tuberculosis and
Binational Health Concerns

For a number of years, tuberculosis has been one of the communicable diseases of most concern to border health officials. This concern is based on the fact that tuberculosis case rates tend to be higher on either side of the border than in most of the interior of each respective country. In addition, tuberculosis is a difficult disease to treat because of the long treatment period (a minimum of 6 months) and the high rate of migration to and from the area. Finally, tuberculosis control is complicated in the border region because of differences in the use of vaccine, diagnostic techniques, treatment regimens, and reporting systems between these two countries.

The administrative and political issues involved with binational tuberculosis control must be viewed within the context of the disease itself. Many of the most contentious issues related to binational cooperation have to do with different methods of tuberculosis control and management. To understand these issues, it is necessary to have a basic understanding of tuberculosis.

Tuberculosis is one of the oldest known diseases of humankind, with traces of the disease having been found in Egyptian mummies. Today, there are approximately 8.8 million new cases of tuberculosis globally per year. Three million people die of the disease each year, and 95% of these cases occur in the developing world (CDC, 1993; World Health Organization, 1995). Until recently, tuberculosis was on a path of steady decline in the developed world. Beginning in 1985, however, the number of tuberculosis cases in the United States and in parts of Europe not only failed to decrease but began to increase. Between 1985 and 1994, the number of tuberculosis cases in the United States increased by 10% (CDC, 1995). In Mexico, tuberculosis case rates were declining beginning with the introduction of antituberculosis drugs in the late 1940s. After the mid-1980s, Mexican tuberculosis rates appear to have leveled off. Between 1988 and 1992, the overall Mexican case rate averaged around 17 per 100,000 population (Direccion General de Epidemiologia, 1993), compared to the U.S. case rate in 1992 of 10.8 per 100,000.

Tuberculosis is spread by a microorganism, *Mycobacterium tuberculosis,* that is carried in droplets in the air. The droplets are formed when a person with active disease coughs, sneezes, laughs, sings, or somehow expels air from the lungs. The bacteria lodge first in the lungs but can spread to the lymph nodes and then other parts of the body through the bloodstream. It is estimated that only 1 out of 10 persons who are infected with the tuberculosis bacillus will develop active disease in his or her lifetime. The chances of developing active disease are greatly increased if a person is coinfected with the HIV virus or if his or her immune system is weakened through other disease or poor nutrition. People who are actively ill with tuberculosis often have a prolonged cough, weakness, weight loss, and fever (American Thoracic Society, 1994; CDC, 1994). Untreated, about one half of patients with tuberculosis will die within 5 years of diagnosis (Brown, 1993).

The first antituberculosis drug, streptomycin, was developed in 1944 and was soon followed by the development of several additional drugs (CDC, 1993; World Health Organization, 1995). There is still no one drug that will eliminate all of the tuberculosis bacillus in any individual. One of the most disturbing aspects of the recent resurgence of tuberculosis is an increase in resistant forms of disease. In each actively infectious person, there are approximately 100 million tuberculosis bacilli, and through natural mutation there are always some of these organisms that are resistant to one or more of the drugs used to treat disease. Resistance develops when an inadequate drug regimen is prescribed or when a patient takes medication erratically for less than the required minimum of 6 months. In either of these two situations, the bacilli that are susceptible to the drugs taken by the patient are killed, leaving a population of resistant bacilli. To eradicate the remaining bacilli, additional and often more expensive and less effective medications are required. In general, patients with multidrug-resistant tuberculosis have a 50% chance of dying from the disease (Tripathy, 1993). The real danger from a public health standpoint is that patients who have developed drug resistance will pass those drug-resistant organisms to other people.

The only test that can detect infection in persons without active disease is the tuberculin skin test, although this test is not totally accurate. The diagnosis of active tuberculosis requires identification of *M. tuberculosis* in specimens from diseased parts of the body. The most common diagnostic specimen is sputum from the lungs. The most frequently used diagnostic technique throughout the developing world, including Mexico, is the smear test. This method "permits only the presumptive diagnosis of TB because [the bacilli] on a smear may be mycobacteria other than *M. tuberculosis,* . . . [and] many TB patients have negative . . . smears" (CDC, 1994, p. 29).

It is a common method for the developing world because it does not require expensive technology. A more reliable but also more expensive method is the sputum culture. This method is necessary to determine if a person has drug-resistant organisms. Chest x-ray examinations will also detect abnormalities that are caused by tuberculosis.

Some of the key issues between the United States and Mexico with regard to binational tuberculosis coordination are related to methods of diagnosis, treatment, prevention, and follow-up. The most significant of these are diagnostic methods, treatment regimens, use of BCG vaccination, and record systems for identifying and following patients.

Currently, only a few laboratories in Mexico have the capability to do culture and drug susceptibility testing on sputum. Mexico follows the World Health Organization recommendations and diagnoses cases using smear testing. This is not unusual or unreasonable, given Mexico's current level of health care resources that can be devoted to laboratories. But the two main disadvantages to using smears instead of culture testing are that some cases will be overlooked and that without culture testing it is impossible to test for the presence of drug resistance.

Closely linked with the issue of culture versus smear testing are discussions over adequate treatment regimens. There are two fundamental differences between the two countries' treatment regimens. The first is that the United States now recommends that in most instances patients should be started on four drugs until drug susceptibilities have been determined, whereas Mexico recommends a three-drug regimen. Second, most of the United States has access to second-line drugs needed to treat drug resistance, whereas most parts of Mexico do not have access to these drugs.

Mexico and the United States are also at odds over the use of BCG vaccination. BCG has never been used routinely in the United States because it has been determined that the vaccine is only useful in high-risk populations in which children are at a greater risk of developing particularly severe forms of tuberculosis. In Mexico, BCG is a component of routine childhood vaccination, and many Mexican health officials feel that the United States is shortsighted in not providing the vaccination to children in high-risk areas. The issue is heightened when U.S. health professionals treat Mexican-born patients because people who have received the BCG vaccination will have a positive tuberculin skin test (Castro, 1994).

The final issue has to do with patient reporting systems. This issue is less contentious but equally difficult to resolve. The development of shared reporting systems between the two countries is invariably one of the key components of binational projects, but it is one of the most difficult to resolve. The two main problems are that the United States and Mexico have different reporting forms and that neither side has developed an effective way to share information on a daily basis (Pan American Health Organization [PAHO], 1993).

These are the main issues for tuberculosis control that affect all binational efforts. Individual areas may have additional unique problems that they must work out as they implement binational projects. Some individual areas may have found solutions for the more global problems presented in this chapter in addition to resolving local issues. These ideas will be further explored in the examination of the two case studies of local binational tuberculosis projects.

Case Studies in
Binational Tuberculosis Control

The two case studies examined here developed between 1991 and 1993. The precedent for these projects was set in 1967, when the CDC established a special Binational Tuberculosis Commission. From 1970 to 1973, a pilot project was initiated in El Paso/Ciudad Juárez that consisted of screening Mexican patients in Ciudad Juárez. Although this project was considered a success, it was determined that there was not a significant amount of transmission of disease, and the program was canceled. Renewed interest in binational cooperation occurred in the late 1980s, largely as a result of the surge in tuberculosis cases in the United States. The first binational project examined here (hereafter referred to as Project 1) was established in 1991 as the first of the "modern" binational tuberculosis projects. The second project (hereafter referred to as Project 2) was established in 1993.

Both projects were established with funding from the CDC. The initial goals of both projects were very similar—namely, (a) to strengthen tuberculosis services on the Mexican side by increasing access to sophisticated laboratory services, treating drug-resistant disease, and increasing outreach efforts; (b) to improve binational referrals/consultations and develop a binational registry; and (c) to increase access to tuberculosis education for health professionals and the community (PAHO, 1993).

Although the projects had similar initial goals, the administration of program activities has differed significantly and ultimately has had a significant effect on the development of each project.

Project 1

Funding for Project 1 comes from the CDC to the Texas Department of Health and is then given to the local health department, which in turn contracts with PAHO to oversee the project in the Mexican sister city. The project is physically housed in the SS offices in the Mexican sister city and staffed by SS personnel.

Much of what has determined the successes and failures of Project 1 has to do with specific characteristics of the local area as well as the relationship between the two sister cities. On the Mexican side, SS, IMSS, and ISSSTE all have a presence. IMSS provides the most bed space, and SS has 81% of the outpatient clinics (Secretaria de Salud, 1993). Both institutions see tuberculosis patients, although the SS is supposed to receive all patient data. Although there is some collaboration between these two institutions in this region, there is not the same degree of cooperation that is seen in some other parts of Mexico.

Project 1 was initially designed to augment existing tuberculosis services provided by the local SS systems in Mexico. Project funds provided by the CDC were to be used to hire additional personnel, improve laboratory services, develop a binational registry, and create educational materials. The program was not designed to operate independently of the Mexican services already in place.

Instead of distributing funds directly to SS, the program was set up to be administered through PAHO. The regional PAHO office was to be responsible for administrative and financial oversight. Although the administrative structures have remained essentially as they were initially designed, certain aspects of the project were altered as the realities of implementation became apparent. One initial flaw in the project was that some of the original staff for the project were chosen by PAHO with little input from the SS. This created initial resistance, and some of the staff eventually had to be replaced. The project also had to contend with personnel changes resulting from changes in political administrations. For Project 1, this meant that the project had to be "resold" to the major health officials in Mexico, and work was delayed.

The design of Project 1 has had a significant effect on the overall outcomes of the project. The fact that Project 1 is linked to the existing Mexican health care structure means that although it is funded through the United States, Mexican health entities exert a fair amount of control over the project. The advantage to this design is that if the project were to disappear tomorrow, there would be less of a void left in its absence. In addition, the project would presumably leave a better educated and equipped staff. The disadvantage in many people's minds is that the current Project 1 design leaves less room for PAHO or local U.S. government input or control. In addition, the project is more open to manipulation by local politics.

Another significant issue regarding Project 1's design is that the program is run through a third agency, PAHO, rather than directly between the two health departments conducting tuberculosis control measures. On one hand, PAHO provides a more global view and has connections with higher-level officials in both countries. On the other hand, the absence of a direct link between the participating local health departments seems to hinder full cooperation between the two health departments. The project becomes less of a binational effort and more of a strengthening of Mexican services.

One final important issue is the lack of coordination among local Mexican health agencies in the region. It is thought by some that the logical link to the local U.S. health department is the SS system because both are charged with delivering services to the indigent population. In Mexico, however, IMSS and ISSSTE are responsible for delivering health care to such a large group of people that it is vital that they be included in any sort of comprehensive attack on tuberculosis.

Project 2

The second binational project (Project 2) developed nearly 2 years after the start of Project 1, with many of the same goals as Project 1 but in a very different political and administrative atmosphere. Project 2's site is in an urban area that is much smaller than Project 1's site. On the Mexican side, IMSS, SS, and ISSSTE each have one general hospital, and SS is responsible for 73% of outpatient clinics. In general, there is a great deal more cooperation between health care agencies, aided by the fact that all major health centers, with the exception of the IMSS hospital, are located in one central area. High-level IMSS, ISSSTE, and SS personnel see one another frequently and often coordinate projects jointly.

In Project 2, unlike Project 1, the local U.S. health department was responsible for administering the binational project in Mexico. PAHO served as a consultant for the early implementation of the project but was not called on to run the project. Another important difference between the two binational projects was the degree of collaboration that occurred among Mexican health agencies in the region. This high level of collaboration was exemplified by the strong binational steering committee brought together for the project.

The project initially intended to serve a coordinating role for all tuberculosis services on the Mexican side, with linkages to the tuberculosis control program on the U.S. side. Soon after it was implemented, this element of the program changed, and day-to-day tuberculosis control activities were taken out of Mexican health entities and administered by Project 2 staff hired specifically by the project. Tuberculosis patients seen by Project 2 staff in Mexico were placed on U.S. treatment regimens and follow-up procedures.

In the short term, Project 2 was very successful in organizing and streamlining tuberculosis services on the Mexican side. However, after approximately a year of operation, the Mexican state government intervened in the project because there was concern about the fact that tuberculosis services had been withdrawn from Mexican health entities and that patients were receiving U.S. treatment regimens. As a result, the project has had to redevelop a number of its services and return tuberculosis control activities to Mexican health agencies.

One of the most positive aspects of Project 2 is the degree of cooperation among Mexican health care agencies. This collaboration allows the project to present a united front and provide a strong set of services to the patient population.

The initial design of Project 2, which consolidated services under local U.S. health department personnel while ensuring short-term success, proved to be a barrier to the long-term advancement of tuberculosis care on the Mexican side. Project 2 had the effect of immediately improving services but eventually weakening tuberculosis control by taking services away from Mexican health entities, rather than trying to strengthen them. Within this design, local Mexican health agencies were not in a position to build the long-term infrastructure needed for the future success of tuberculosis control, particularly once the funding from CDC necessarily decreases.

Conclusions

From the preceding analysis, four general recommendations emerge for future projects. The first is that future projects should allow for more binational input during the planning and early implementation stages. Project 1 and Project 2, though involving both sides to a certain extent, were largely based on the design presented by policy makers in the United States. One way to ensure greater binational planning would be for funding agencies to provide a pool of money to a binational organization such as the U.S.-Mexico Border Health Association (USMBHA). To receive funds, participating organizations would be required to demonstrate that the proposed projects had been planned with significant input from both sides. Such an arrangement, even if all available funding originally came from the United States, would eliminate some of the political issues surrounding the development and implementation of binational projects with U.S. money and control.

The second recommendation is that the U.S. and Mexico reach an agreement on treatment, laboratory work, and BCG vaccinations for the border area. This is an issue that local areas can influence, but ultimately the agreement will have to take place on a national level within both countries. It is not necessary for the United States and Mexico to implement the same treatment and diagnostic procedures on a national level, but in the border region, with its shared population, the two sides should attempt to standardize where possible.

The third recommendation is that, as much as possible, agencies within each country should coordinate services. Clearly tuberculosis control will improve in both the United States and Mexico with greater internal collaboration. If each country cannot provide a unified front internally, it will be that much more difficult to engage in effective binational collaboration.

The fourth recommendation is that, wherever possible, future projects should work within existing public health structures unless the project is creating a new entity that is expected to last well beyond the duration of the project. Even though it is easier to remove and isolate program activities to gain control over them, in the long run, such actions may result in weak programs. Future projects should work to improve and coordinate existing services rather than isolate them.

Overall, both Project 1 and Project 2 have been very successful in achieving the first stage of binational cooperation between the United

States and Mexico in tuberculosis control. Project planners in both areas fully intend to carry on the learning process and to continually improve program activities.

References

American Thoracic Society and Centers for Disease Control and Prevention. (1994). Treatment of TB and TB infection in adults and children. *American Journal of Respiratory and Critical Care Medicine, 149,* 1369-1374.

Brown, P. (1993). A disease that is alive and kicking. *World Health, 46*(4), 4-5.

Castro, K. (1994, January). *U.S. strategies for tuberculosis control: A focus on the Mexican immigrants.* Paper presented at the U.S.-Mexico Border Tuberculosis Review Meeting, El Paso, TX.

Centers for Disease Control and Prevention. (1993). Estimates of global tuberculosis morbidity and mortality. *Morbidity and Mortality Weekly Report, 42,* 961-964.

Centers for Disease Control and Prevention. (1994). *Core curriculum on tuberculosis.* Atlanta: Author.

Centers for Disease Control and Prevention. (1995). *Tuberculosis statistics in the United States, 1994.* Atlanta: Author.

Direccion General de Epidemiologia. (1993). *Annual statistical report on tuberculosis.* Mexico City, Mexico: Secretaria de Salud Publica.

General Accounting Office. (1988). *Health care: Availability in the Texas-Mexico border area* (HRD-89-12). Washington, DC: Author.

Gonzales-Block, M. A. (1993). *Las politicas de salud en la frontera Mexico-Estados Unidos.* Unpublished manuscript, Colegia de la Frontera Norte, Tijuana, Mexico.

Jacquart, K. (1994). *U.S. public health services.* Unpublished manuscript for North American Free Trade Agreement and Health Care Policy Research Project, Lyndon B. Johnson School of Public Affairs.

Lopez Acuña, D. (1980). Health services in Mexico. *Journal of Public Health Policy, 1*(1), 83-95.

Office of the Governor. (1993). *Health and human services issues along the U.S.-Mexico border in Texas and Mexico* (Rep. No. 93-0325). Austin, TX: Author.

Pan American Health Organization. (1993). *Tuberculosis control program: A binational approach, program review.* El Paso, TX: Author.

Rodriguez, V. (1992). Mexico's decentralization in the 1980s: Promises, promises, promises. In A. Morris & S. Lowder (Eds.), *Decentralization in Latin America: An evaluation.* New York: Praeger.

Samuels, B. (1992). *Public health system in Texas* (Working Paper No. 66). Austin, TX: Lyndon B. Johnson School of Public Affairs.

Secretaria de Salud. (1993). *Annuario estadistico 1992.* Mexico, D.F.: Author.

Soberon, G., Valdez, C., & de Caso, O. (1989). La salud sin fronteras y las fronteras en la salud. *Salud Publica de Mexico, 31,* 813-822.

Tripathy, S. P. (1993). Multidrug-resistant tuberculosis. *World Health, 46*(4), 19.

Ward, P. (1986). *Welfare politics in Mexico*. London: Allen & Unwin.

World Health Organization. (1995). Global epidemiology of tuberculosis: Morbidity and mortality of a worldwide epidemic. *Journal of the American Medical Association, 273,* 220-226.

Chapter 7

‿✦‿

A PATCH FOR THE QUILT

HIV/AIDS, Homosexual Men, and Community Mobilization on the U.S.-Mexico Border

JESUS RAMIREZ-VALLES
MARC A. ZIMMERMAN
ENRIQUE SUAREZ
GRACIELA DE LA ROSA

This chapter describes and analyzes an HIV/AIDS community-based education project among homosexual men conducted in the border city of Ciudad Juárez, Mexico. It includes a brief review of the epidemiology of HIV/AIDS and unsafe sex among Mexican homosexual males and community-based interventions among this population. It also describes an empowering approach for community-based education, including a description of the project and evaluation. In this section, we emphasize the recruiting, training, and activities of homosexual male health promoters involved in the intervention. The evaluation includes both quantitative and qualitative data. We conclude with a discussion of the implications for community-based interventions among this population on the Mexico-U.S. border. The need for cooperative efforts between the United States and Mexico to prevent the spread of HIV/AIDS is discussed.

"The U.S.-Mexico border *es una herida abierta* where the Third World grates against the first and bleeds. And before a scab forms it hemorrhages again, the lifeblood of two worlds merging to form a third country—a border culture" (Anzaldua, 1987, p. 3).

More than a decade after the first AIDS case was reported in Mexico, homosexual and bisexual men[1] are still the most vulnerable group for HIV infection (Izazola-Licea, Avila-Figueroa, Gortmaker, & del Rio-Chiriboga, 1995; Pan American Health Organization, 1992). In Mexico, the number of cases due to unprotected male-to-male sexual practices continues to increase (EPI-CONASIDA, 1992; Izazola-Licea et al., 1995). It is estimated that 75% of the 19,090 AIDS cases reported are associated with male-to-male sexual practices (Izazola-Licea et al., 1995). More than half of these cases are in the age group 25 to 44 years (EPI-CONASIDA, 1992). These statistics, however, are only the tip of the iceberg because many cases are unreported and because many of the male-to-male sex-related cases are reported by the individuals as heterosexual transmission (EPI-CONASIDA, 1992).

In the United States, Mexican American homosexual men (and Hispanic homosexual men in general) are similarly affected. The AIDS prevalence among Hispanic homosexual and bisexual males is one of the highest of the United States (Centers for Disease Control and Prevention [CDC], 1991; Singer et al., 1990). Researchers have reported that this group has a higher incidence of unprotected sex than whites and African Americans (Doll et al., 1991; Jimenez, McKirnan, & LaBoy, 1990; Linn et al., 1989). Through 1995, 51% of AIDS cases among adults and adolescents in the United States were attributed to sex between men (CDC, 1995). Of the 73,669 cases reported among Hispanics through 1995, 44% were attributed to sex between men (CDC, 1995). In 1995, 1,027 AIDS cases were reported among Hispanics identified as born in Mexico, and over half (54%) of these cases were attributed to sex between men (CDC, 1995).

The most common causes for the high prevalence of HIV and AIDS among Mexican and Mexican American homosexual men are unprotected receptive anal intercourse and multiple sexual partners (Lemp et al., 1994; St. Lawrence, Hood, Brasfield, & Kelly, 1989). Several researchers have documented that Mexican and Mexican American men who have sex with men tend to practice more anal intercourse than other forms of sex and that they expect to obtain sexual satisfaction from anal intercourse rather than fellatio (Almaguer, 1991; Alonso & Koreck, 1989; Caceres, Gotuzzo, Wignall, & Campos, 1991; Carrier, 1976; Magana & Carrier, 1991). Studies among Mexican homosexuals have found that a history of receptive anal sex, mixed sexual behavior (both insertive and receptive anal intercourse), multiple sexual partners, and a history of sexually transmitted diseases are associated with HIV infection (Garcia Garcia et al., 1991; Guerena-Burgueno, Benenson, & Sepulveda, 1991; Izazola-Licea et al., 1991, 1995). These researchers also reported that less than 30% of the homosexual and bisexual men had used condoms in their last sexual encounter. Yet Izazola-Licea et al. (1995) found that only condom use in all sexual encounters was a protective factor against HIV.

This epidemic has generated community mobilization among homosexual men in Mexico as in other areas of the world. Community-based groups, governments, and nongovernmental organizations (NGOs) have undertaken prevention programs for homosexual males in Mexico and other Latin American countries (Carrier, 1995; Carrillo, 1994; Diaz, 1995; Figueroa, 1990; Sepulveda, 1992). Nonetheless, few of them go beyond informing participants about the mechanics of AIDS prevention (Caceres et al., 1991; Carrillo, 1994; Lumsden, 1991; Mott, Moreira, Ribeiro, Badaro, & Johnson, 1990). Researchers have pointed out, however, that multiple activities on a continuous basis are a more effective HIV/AIDS educational approach than the sole provision of information at one point in time (Levine, 1991; Zimmerman, Janz, & Wren, 1995). In this chapter, we describe and analyze a community-based HIV/AIDS prevention program for homosexual men in Ciudad Juárez, Mexico, a border city with El Paso, Texas. First, we describe the border context in which this project took place. Second, we present the community empowerment approach used for developing, implementing, and evaluating the program. Third, we describe the project activities and evaluation. Finally, we discuss the implications of the project with regard to efforts to prevent the spread of HIV and AIDS along the Mexico-U.S. border.

The Border

Mexican homosexual men living in northern border cities, such as Tijuana and Ciudad Juárez, are at increased risk for HIV infection due to frequent contact with men in the United States (Izazola-Licea et. al., 1991; Sepulveda, 1992). They may receive the influence of different patterns of sexual practices from the non-Hispanic white homosexual population, which could increase the risk of infection. Among the non-Hispanic white homosexual male population, anal and oral mixed sex behavior is a dominant pattern, whereas among Mexican men, the pattern tends to be single role, either receptive or insertive anal sex[2] (Almaguer, 1991; Carrier, 1995;

Magana & Carrier, 1991). In addition, the migration from Mexico to the United States is concentrated in states with high seroprevalence, California and Texas (Bronfman, Camposortega, & Medina, 1989; Sepulveda, 1992). In Tijuana, for instance, HIV seroprevalence among homosexual and bisexual men ranges from 6.8% to 11.6%, and condom use ranges from 26% to 45.9% (Guerena-Burgueno et al., 1991; Izazola-Licea et al., 1991). El Paso has reported 551 AIDS cases through 1995 (CDC, 1995). Comparable data are not available for Ciudad Juárez.

The Mexico-U.S. border is best described by its permeability/impermeability. Ciudad Juárez and El Paso, although separated by a legal national border, share an economy, a labor force, and a culture (Martinez, 1994). The population of this international community is about 1.5 million. Ciudad Juárez is characterized by its large population of immigrants from southern Mexico. Immigrants come here either to enter into the United States or to work in Ciudad Juárez's large *maquiladora* industry. In El Paso, almost 70% of the population is of Mexican origin, and the majority of the population speak both Spanish and English (Martinez, 1994). Thousands of residents on both sides of the border commute every day for work, commerce, and family and entertainment activities (Bringas, 1995). This social dynamic is also evident in the homosexual community. Gay entertainment and gathering areas in both cities are within walking distance of one another. Residents on both sides of the border frequent the same places in both cities. Similarly, intimate relations and social networks extend to both cities. The social blending in this international border region nonetheless coexists with class, race, and sexual identity differences and conflicts (Martinez, 1994; Vila, 1995). Its homosexual community mirrors this paradox.

In the late 1980s in the El Paso/Ciudad Juárez area, several governmental, private, and community-based organizations started working in HIV/AIDS prevention. They focused their work on intravenous drug users, female sex workers, and homosexual men, but with little coordination in their efforts. In Ciudad Juárez, as in other Mexican cities, a small group of homosexual men began looking for resources (e.g., condoms and brochures) on both sides of the border to do small-scale educational work in the homosexual community. In their search, they came into contact with the Mexican Federation of Private Associations for Community Development (FEMAP), which had initiated an HIV/AIDS prevention program with female sex workers. FEMAP is an NGO with 20 years of experience in community-based health programs in Mexico. FEMAP's approach is based on the recruitment and training of community members as health promoters (see, e.g., Kirsch, Andrade, Osterling, Sherwood-Fabre, & Galvan, 1995). Consequently, a group of homosexual men collaborated with FEMAP to develop and implement a community-based education program for homosexual men. This collaboration developed from FEMAP's philosophy of community participation, using empowerment as the guiding theory.

Empowerment Theory

Health education programs are frequently based on a professional client relationship. In these types of relationships, dependence on the professional is encouraged, and people are assumed to be passive and in need of help (Zimmerman, in press). Alternatively, Freire (1970) presented an approach referred to as *empowerment education.* In this method, professionals work collaboratively with participants to promote participation and control. This approach employs group dialogue and work to increase social consciousness and social action to solve problems. Empowerment educational processes have been used in many health-related programs, including substance abuse prevention (Wallerstein & Bernstein, 1988), women's health in rural areas (Minkler & Cox, 1980), and social support for the impoverished elderly (Minkler, 1985).

The HIV/AIDS prevention program developed by FEMAP and the group of homosexual men used an empowerment approach. Zimmerman (1995) posited that the process dimension of empowerment theory refers to designing interventions that enable individuals to develop and practice skills and to influence their sociopolitical environment. Empowering processes are by definition contextually based and social change oriented. They consist of a collective learning process based on the interconnection between the development of awareness and action (Cornell Empowerment Group, 1989; Freire, 1970; Mechanic, 1991; Rappaport, 1984). An empowerment education process may therefore influence individuals' health-related behavior by enhancing their perceived control and self-efficacy and increasing their understanding of the agents that may facilitate or inhibit the capacity to be proactive in their efforts to improve their own health and the health of their community (Zimmerman, 1995).

An empowering education starts by involving those for whom it is intended (i.e., participants) in its development, implementation, and evaluation (Wallerstein, 1992; Zimmerman, 1995, in press). The process begins by identifying and working with community leaders. Next, it assists people in developing skills so they can become less dependent on professionals (Kelly, 1971; Wallerstein, 1992; Zimmerman, 1995). These might include decision making, problem solving, data collection and analysis, or resource mobilization skills. The educational process promotes a context for people to work together in making decisions and generating action (Maton & Salem, 1995).

The Project

The intervention was the first attempt ever made in the homosexual community in Ciudad Juárez to develop a community-based HIV/AIDS prevention program. It started when FEMAP and two homosexual men who were very involved in the community joined forces. These two men were invited by FEMAP to develop a community-based program. They were named coordinators of the program. Both coordinators received training from FEMAP staff on HIV/AIDS, community assessment, participant recruitment, and group facilitation. The basic intervention and evaluation plans were developed collaboratively by the organization staff and the two community members. The project was designed to allow participants to shape it in ways that they believed were most appropriate. The program was fundamentally created to reduce the risk for HIV infection due to sexual transmission among Mexican homosexual and bisexual males living in Ciudad Juárez. Its primary objectives were to promote safe sex practices among participants and to involve them as voluntary health promoters in the community.

Needs Assessment

The first phase of the intervention was to obtain information about the HIV/AIDS attitudes, knowledge, and behaviors in the Ciudad Juárez homosexual community. This phase was also designed to be a first step to recruit and involve a broad group of individuals from the community to participate in the program development. Fifteen members of the community were recruited by the two coordinators to help with this needs assessment. The assessment included face-to-face interviews with 200 individuals and focus group discussions with 30 community members. Information collected in this assessment was also used as pretest data to compare with results from a posttest survey a year later to evaluate the program. Ramirez, Suarez, De la Rosa, Castro, and Zimmerman (1994) described the procedure and results of the needs assessment in greater detail.

The 15 volunteers helped develop the interview protocol and sampling strategy. They also conducted the interviews. The two coordinators trained the 15 volunteers in interviewing skills and provided basic HIV/AIDS information to them. The 30 participants in the focus groups were recruited from friends and acquaintances of the coordinators and the 15 interviewers. Two focus group discussions were conducted by the coordinators and stressed health in general, homosexuality, and HIV/AIDS risk behaviors.

Survey respondents (all males) were approached in several settings (e.g., homes, workplaces, streets, parks, and bars). The interview protocol assessed sociodemographic data, HIV/AIDS knowledge, condom use and attitudes, and sexual practices. All respondents were residents of Ciudad Juárez. Two thirds ($n = 133$) self-identified as gay, 29% ($n = 58$) as bisexual, and 2% ($n = 5$) as transvestites. Their mean age was 26 years. The majority of the respondents (74%; $n = 149$) had lived in Ciudad Juárez for at least 5 years, 80% ($n = 160$) had at least completed secondary education, and 95% ($n = 190$) were employed.

Analyses of the data revealed that although individuals were knowledgeable about HIV/AIDS, they had not translated this knowledge into safe sexual practices. Respondents had over four sexual partners in the previous month, and over half had mixed anal (58%) or mixed oral (59%) sex. They averaged 65% condom use in the last 10 sexual relations, and condom use during high-risk sex practices (i.e., anal insertive or receptive intercourse) occurred only 60% of the time. Factory workers and individuals who met sexual partners in the streets had more sexual partners. Less condom use was found among older respondents, individuals with a higher number of sex partners, and individuals having negative attitudes toward condom use. These results are consistent with those of other researchers who have studied similar populations (Izazola-Licea et al., 1991, 1995).

Every interview respondent and participant in the focus groups was invited to attend regular weekly sessions to learn more about HIV/AIDS prevention and to begin to plan a community intervention. The purpose of the sessions was to enhance safe sex practices and to prepare a cadre of volunteer health promoters to provide HIV/AIDS education in the community. A total of 37 individuals volunteered to participate in the weekly group sessions. These 37 participants and the 15 interviewers worked together to plan and implement educational activities in the community in their role as health promoters.

Health Promoters' Educational Sessions

The weekly sessions lasted approximately 3 hours each and took place over an 8-month period. These sessions were designed to provide HIV/AIDS information through group discussions, train participants as health promoters, and plan outreach and community activities. They were also used for team building and mutual support. Details on this process are presented elsewhere (Zimmerman, Ramirez-Valles, Suarez, De la Rosa, & Castro, 1997).

The initial weekly meetings were devoted primarily to education on HIV and AIDS. These sessions were designed as group discussions in which participants and staff took turns facilitating. Participants discussed and voted on topics to be covered, as well as ideas for the role of the group in providing HIV/AIDS education in the community. Topics covered included HIV risk behaviors, safe sex, HIV testing, self-esteem, substance abuse, HIV/AIDS treatment alternatives, and other sexually transmitted diseases. Group discussions also provided participants an opportunity to share their concerns and experiences. They often talked about "coming out" processes, identity development, fears about testing, and access to health services. The results of the needs assessment were presented and discussed with participants during these sessions to help plan their activities.

Participants and staff members employed several group techniques to maintain a participatory learning process. Participants learned about communication with partners relating to safe sex practices through role-playing activities. Participants worked together on strategies to reach people in bars and distribute condoms through problem-solving processes. Videos featuring testimonies and HIV/AIDS and drug abuse information were also used to facilitate discussion. Participants were given printed educational and informational materials to use as reference material and to pass on to other people. Several sessions were devoted to special workshops given by outside experts from Mexico and the United States on sexuality, providing support to people with AIDS (PWAs), and safe sex practices. These experts were identified and recruited by both staff and participants.

Subsequent sessions were dedicated to training participants to be community health promoters. The training focused on the specific tasks to be accomplished by health promoters: outreach, condom distribution, and face-to-face education. At the end of their training as health promoters, a graduation was held in which each participant was given a diploma. This celebration not only helped acknowledge participants' accomplishment but also helped motivate them.

Health promoters distributed educational materials and condoms in bars, streets, and workplaces; referred individuals to social services and medical institutions; distributed information about HIV/AIDS; and invited participants to attend their weekly discussion sessions. Health promoters also documented their activities by recording the number of condoms they distributed, the number of presentations given, and the number of referrals made. Five of these health promoters became leaders for groups of the remaining health promoters. Their duties included ensuring that the health promoters were equipped with condoms and educational materials to distribute, arranging community presentations, and maintaining the health promoters' record keeping. In this work, the tasks of the staff were to help assess the obstacles and opportunities that health promoters faced, to join them in their outreach work, to maintain their enthusiasm and motivation, and to continue training them on an individual basis. These staff activities were on a one-to-one basis with each health promoter in addition to the weekly group discussions.

As the group developed over time, several discussions centered on community activities that participants could do to further their goal of HIV/AIDS prevention. The activities discussed were solely the result of initiatives taken by the participants. The activities focused on broader social change, resource mobilization, and community consciousness-raising about AIDS and related issues. These activities are described below in the evaluation section.

Evaluation

Zimmerman et al. (1997) described the procedure and the results of the evaluation of the health promoters model employed in this project. A pretest-posttest design compared individual changes on HIV/AIDS knowledge, number of sexual partners, and condom use between health promoters and a comparison group formed by individuals who received information from health promoters. Participant observation data were also collected to assess the community activities that the group engaged in.

Individual-Level Outcomes

Data were collected before the intervention and again 12 months later. Both pretest and posttest interviews were conducted by the 15 gay male interviewers described above. Individuals who decided to participate in the weekly group sessions were considered to be participants (i.e., health promoters) in the intervention ($n = 37$). Nonparticipants were considered to be those individuals who had received information from participants in their work as health promoters and for whom pre- and posttest data were available ($n = 55$). Four individual-level outcomes were assessed: HIV/AIDS knowledge, number of sexual partners in the previous month, condom use in the last 10 sexual encounters, and frequency of condom use during high-risk sexual practices (i.e., anal insertive intercourse, anal receptive intercourse, and oral sex).

Zimmerman et al. (1997) found no differences between the comparison and intervention groups for number of sexual partners in the previous month. Intervention participants, however, reported more HIV/AIDS knowledge, more condom use in the last 10 sexual encounters, and greater frequency of condom use during high-risk sexual practices than nonparticipants. These results suggest that the involvement of individuals in this educational process helped them to increase their safe sex practices.

Community-Level Outcomes

Qualitative information about participants' activities in the community was also gathered. This information was collected through informal conversations during the project with participants and staff. Participant observation of weekly discussion sessions, outreach activities, and community activities was also conducted. Similar observations and informal conversations were conducted a year after the funding of the project ended.

In their role as health promoters, participants worked in pairs in bars, parks, and streets. They mostly worked on weekends to distribute condoms and educational pamphlets and to put up posters in bars. Health promoters also distributed condoms in steambaths and at workplaces (e.g., *maquiladora* plants). In essence, they made their role as health promoters an integrated part of their daily lives. They became recognized by members of the community as knowledgeable and trustworthy about HIV/AIDS issues. The level of commitment of the health promoters is notable in light of the sometimes hostile social environment that homosexual men face. Their outreach work implied many risks, such as harassment by bar patrons and the police. For example, police in Ciudad Juárez are known to conduct raids in bars and to cruise areas frequented by homosexuals. Although none of the health promoters were detained by the police, several health promoters in FEMAP's program with female sex workers were arrested while distributing condoms in the streets.

Health promoters also carried out several community activities beyond the distribution of condoms and educational dissemination. Many of their activities were supported by FEMAP and other agencies on both sides of the border. Health promoters were able to mobilize material resources, such as medicines, educational brochures, and small amounts of funding. They also conducted their own fund-raising activities (e.g., donations, contests) to help people with HIV/AIDS.

As participants became aware of the large number of AIDS cases in the city and the reluctance of health professionals to receive HIV and AIDS patients, they developed strategies to address these issues. They went to private and public health service agencies and hospitals to advocate for AIDS patients. They met formally with officials, administrators, and physicians to discuss the problems experienced by patients (e.g., accessibility of services, treatment, and medication). They also addressed health care personnel fears and concerns about treating PWAs. Health administrators then invited health promoters to provide suggestions for HIV/AIDS prevention and care to health care personnel.

Participants also created a support system to provide assistance to PWAs. They were referred to FEMAP by hospitals and HIV testing agencies. Support was provided on an individual basis. Coordinators linked PWAs to a health promoter. This strategy was used to ensure confidentiality, given that many PWAs did not want their identity revealed. Health promoters helped the PWAs to obtain whatever assistance they wanted (e.g., financial assistance, food, and medicines).

Health promoters created an informal network of resources with agencies and groups in Ciudad Juárez and El Paso to develop and sustain their activities. Consequently, they connected agencies on both sides of the border to acknowledge several public events (e.g., AIDS World Day). Health promoters also learned about the AIDS quilt tradition in the United States and made a quilt to remember those lives taken by AIDS in Ciudad Juárez. The quilt was exhibited in El Paso.

Many of the health promoters' community activities continued after the funding of the program ended. Several of the participants continue to distribute condoms, refer individuals to health and social services, care for people with HIV and AIDS, and organize educational presentations. Some of them have joined other organizations and have continued their HIV/AIDS prevention activities in that context. Other participants, especially those who were the most involved, decreased their level of involvement due to the stress encountered. They were simply burned out after 2 years of hard and often painful work.

A Patch for the Quilt

This case study provides an example of how an empowering process may be effective in promoting HIV/AIDS preventive behavior and community mobilization among homosexual men on the Mexico-U.S. border. The educational process was empowering because it provided participants with opportunities to participate in decision making about the intervention and to take ownership of it. It maintained a participatory approach in that participants and staff shared leadership. They worked together to define the program, identify community resources, implement their plans, and evaluate their efforts. The program helped participants increase their awareness of the resources available, as well as the institutional barriers and the means to overcome them. The program also assisted participants in developing knowledge and skills necessary to provide HIV/AIDS education, collect relevant information, and conduct effective outreach activities. This case study, in sum, illustrates how "a good process of mobilization and organizing results in learning from the very process and goes beyond" (Freire, quoted in Bell, Gaventa, & Peters, 1990, p. 117).

Empowerment education, as a patch for a quilt, may be an especially effective approach to prevent the spread of HIV/AIDS among homosexual men on the Mexico-U.S. border. This approach underscores the collaborative role of health educators, which allows community members to take control over the design and implementation of the program. Community members have intimate knowledge and understanding of the sexual practices and norms in their community, more insight about effective strategies to change risk behavior, and a better rapport in communicating with their peers on both sides of the border. They may also be more competent in recognizing and confronting issues such as differences in class, race, and sexual identity. In addition, they may be more knowledgeable about activities, resource networks, and community leaders on both sides of the border. In the case presented here, the empowerment approach enabled participants to use the permeability of the border as they developed informal supportive ties with groups and organizations in El Paso. Empowerment education may also help build a formal coordination of efforts on the Mexico-U.S. border—a missing patch—to address HIV/AIDS.

The impermeability of the border, however, is one of the factors that may hinder the extension of empowerment education effects. Coordination of efforts among NGOs, service agencies, and government agencies in Ciudad Juárez/El Paso has been difficult. These different groups often are engaged in competition, partly due to the way that public institutions and private foundations allocate financial resources. NGOs are forced to compete among themselves and with government agencies for financial resources, human resources (e.g., volunteers and professionals), and geographic areas of work. Although over the years several efforts to coordinate activities within and between Ciudad Juárez and El Paso have been undertaken, they have failed to generate a sustained coordination. These difficulties are often fueled by class, race/ethnicity, and nationality divisions among homosexual men. In Mexico, NGOs and grassroots groups face extreme financial constraints that make their work difficult to sustain (Carrillo, 1994; Diaz, 1995; Hernandez, 1995). In the United States, however, NGOs and grassroots groups have been more successful in attracting funds and maintaining their programs.

Homosexual men in El Paso are better organized than their counterparts in Ciudad Juárez and are better equipped to initiate and promote collaboration with their peers south of the Rio Grande. An empowerment approach in Ciudad Juárez helped provide a motivated and organized counterpart to the well-financed and supported El Paso HIV/AIDS prevention and service activities. Empowering strategies help to motivate volunteers, build community competence, and enhance resources for prevention of HIV/AIDS. Community-based activities may be a vital way to reduce both the social and political barriers formed by an international border. Mexico and the United States are equally responsible for the prevention of HIV/AIDS along their border. The Mexican homosexual community mobilization efforts discussed in this case study have added a patch to the quilt of HIV/AIDS prevention.

Notes

1. The use of categories such as *homosexual, bisexual,* and *gay* in this context is particularly difficult, given their different and diverse social and cultural meanings and uses. The investigation and understanding of these social categories are central to HIV/AIDS prevention but are beyond the scope of this chapter. For general discussions on the topic, see Almaguer (1991), Carrier (1976), and Murray (1995). We will use the terms *homosexual, gay,* and *bisexual* interchangeably.

2. These behavioral patterns are generalizations that should not be substituted for actual individual variations. As Murray (1995) observed, "Behavior and (sexual) identity are more complex in messy reality" (p. 51).

References

Almaguer, T. (1991). Chicano men: A cartography of homosexual identity and behavior. *Differences, 3,* 79-96.

Alonso, A., & Koreck, M. (1989). Silences: "Hispanics," AIDS, and sexual practices. *Differences, 1,* 101-124.

Anzaldua, G. (1987). *Borderlands/La frontera: The new mestiza.* San Francisco: Aunt Lute.

Bell, B., Gaventa, J., & Peters, J. (Eds.). (1990). *We make the road by walking: Conversations on education and social change: Myles Horton and Paulo Freire.* Philadelphia: Temple University Press.

Bringas, R. (1995). Frontera y turismo o las fronteras del turismo. In P. Gondard & J. Revel-Mouroz (Eds.), *La frontiere Mexique-Etats-Unis: Mutations economiques, sociales et territoriales* (pp. 289-307). Paris: Editions de L'iheal.

Bronfman, M., Camposortega, S., & Medina, H. (1989). Myths and realities of the migration-AIDS relationship: The case of Mexican migration to the United States [Abstract]. *V International Conference on AIDS, 5,* 893.

Caceres, C., Gotuzzo, E., Wignall, S., & Campos, M. (1991). Sexual behavior and frequency of antibodies to type 1 human immunodeficiency virus (HIV-1) in a group of Peruvian male homosexuals. *Bulletin of the Panamerican Health Organization, 25,* 306-311.

Carrier, J. (1976). Cultural factors affecting urban Mexican male homosexual behavior. *Archives of Sexual Behavior, 5,* 103-124.

Carrier, J. (1995). *De los otros: Intimacy and homosexuality among Mexican men.* New York: Columbia University Press.

Carrillo, H. (1994). Another crack in the mirror: The politics of AIDS prevention in Mexico. *International Quarterly of Community Health Education, 14,* 129-152.

Centers for Disease Control and Prevention. (1991, October). *HIV/AIDS Surveillance Report.* Atlanta: Author.

Centers for Disease Control and Prevention. (1995, June). *HIV/AIDS Surveillance Report.* Atlanta: Author.

Cornell Empowerment Group. (1989). Empowerment and family support. *Networking Bulletin, 1,* pp. 1-23.

Diaz, G. (1995). Rasquese con sus propias unas: Organizaciones no gubernamentales de lucha contra el SIDA. *Fem, 19,* 4-9.

Doll, L., Byers, R., Bolan, G., Douglas, J., Moss, P., Weller, P., Joy, D., Barthlow, B., & Harrison, J. (1991). Homosexual men who engage in high risk sexual behavior. *Journal of Sexually Transmitted Diseases, 18,* 170-175.

EPI-CONASIDA. (1992, May). *SIDA/ETS Boletin Mensual, 5.*

Figueroa, A. (1990). *Mexico, participacion civil en la lucha contra el SIDA: Catalogo de organizaciones no gubernamentales e instituciones de educacion superior.* Mexico, D.F.

Freire, P. (1970). *Pedagogy of the oppressed.* New York: Seabury.

Garcia Garcia, M., Valdespino, J., Izazola, J., Palacios, M., & Sepulveda, J. (1991). Bisexuality in Mexico: Current perspectives. In R. Tielman, M. Carballo, & A. Hendriks (Eds.), *Bisexuality and AIDS: A global perspective* (pp. 41-58). Buffalo, NY: Prometheus.

Guerena-Burgueno, F., Benenson, A., & Sepulveda, J. (1991). HIV-1 prevalence in selected Tijuana sub-populations. *American Journal of Public Health, 81,* 623-625.

Hernandez, J. (1995). Confronting reality: A personal perspective on the first decade of HIV prevention. In Y. Shiokawa & T. Kitamura (Eds.), *Global challenge of AIDS: Ten years of HIV/AIDS research* (pp. 298-302). Tokyo: Kodansha.

Izazola-Licea, J., Avila-Figueroa, R., Gortmaker, S., & del Rio-Chiriboga, C. (1995). Transmision homosexual del VIH/SIDA en Mexico. *Salud Publica de Mexico, 37,* 602-614.

Izazola-Licea, J., Valdespino-Gomez, J., Gortmaker, S., Townsend, J., Becker, J., Palacios-Martinez, M., Mueller, N., & Sepulveda, J. (1991). HIV-1 seropositivity and behavioral sociological risks among homosexual and bisexual men in six Mexican cities. *Journal of Acquired Immune Deficiency Syndrome, 4,* 614-622.

Jimenez, D., McKirnan, D. J., & LaBoy, F. (1990). Social settings and AIDS-risk sexual behavior among inner-city minority [Abstract]. *VII International Conference on AIDS, 6,* 258.

Kelly, J. (1971). Qualities for the community psychologist. *American Psychologist, 26,* 897-903.

Kirsch, H., Andrade, S., Osterling, J., Sherwood-Fabre, L., & Galvan, A. (1995). Empowerment, participation, and prevention: Use of the community promoter model in northern Mexico. In H. Kirsch (Ed.), *Drug lessons and education programs in developing countries* (pp. 179-194). New Brunswick, NJ: Transaction.

Lemp, G., Hirozawa, A., Givertz, D., Nieri, G., Anderson, L., Lindegren, M., Janssen, R., & Katz, M. (1994). Seroprevalence of HIV and risk behaviors among young homosexual and bisexual men. *Journal of the American Medical Association, 272,* 449-454.

Levine, C. (1991). AIDS prevention and education: Reframing the message. *AIDS Education and Prevention, 3,* 147-163.

Linn, L., Spiegel, S., Mathews, W., Leake, B., Lien, R., & Brook, S. (1989). Recent sexual behaviors among homosexual men seeking primary medical care. *Archives of Internal Medicine, 142,* 2685-2690.

Lumsden, I. (1991). *Homosexualidad, sociedad, y estado en Mexico.* (L. Zapata, Trans.). Mexico, D.F.: Solediciones Colectivo Sol.

Magana, J., & Carrier, J. (1991). Mexican and Mexican American male sexual behavior and spread of AIDS in California. *Journal of Sex Research, 28,* 425-441.

Martinez, O. (1994). *Border people: Life and society in the U.S.-Mexico borderlands.* Tucson: University of Arizona Press.

Maton, K., & Salem, D. (1995). Organizational characteristics of empowering community settings: A multiple case study approach. *American Journal of Community Psychology, 23,* 631-656.

Mechanic, D. (1991, February). *Adolescents at risk: New directions.* Paper presented at the Seventh Annual Conference on Health Policy, Ithaca, NY.

Minkler, M. (1985). Building supportive ties and sense of community among inner-city elderly: The Tenderloin Senior Outreach Project. *Health Education Quarterly, 12,* 303-314.

Minkler, M., & Cox, K. (1980). Creating critical consciousness in health: Applications of Freire's philosophy and methods to the health care setting. *International Journal of Health Services, 10,* 311-322.

Mott, L., Moreira, E., Ribeiro, T., Badaro, R., & Johnson, W. (1990). Impact of condom use to prevent HIV transmission among male homosexuals in Bahia, Brazil [Abstract]. *VII International Conference on AIDS, 6,* 3075.

Murray, S. (1995). *Latin American homosexualities.* Albuquerque: University of New Mexico Press.

Panamerican Health Organization. (1992). *Las condiciones de salud en las Americas* (Vol. 1). Washington, DC.

Ramirez, J., Suarez, E., De la Rosa, G., Castro, M., & Zimmerman, M. (1994). AIDS knowledge and sexual behavior among Mexican gay and bisexual males. *AIDS Education and Prevention, 6,* 163-174.

Rappaport, J. (1984). Studies in empowerment: Introduction to the issue. *Prevention in Human Services, 3,* 1-7.

Sepulveda, J. (1992). Prevention through information and education: Experience from Mexico. In J. Sepulveda, H. Feneberg, & J. Mann (Eds.), *AIDS prevention through education: A world view* (pp. 127-144). New York: Oxford University Press.

Singer, M., Flores, C., Davison, L., Burke, G., Castillo, Z., Scalon, K., & Rivera, M. (1990). SIDA: The economic, social, and cultural context of AIDS among Latinos. *Medical Anthropology Quarterly, 4,* 72-114.

St. Lawrence, J., Hood, H., Brasfield, T., & Kelly, J. (1989). Differences in gay men's AIDS risk knowledge and behavior patterns in high and low AIDS prevalence cities. *Public Health Reports, 104,* 391-395.

Vila, P. (1995, August). *The employment of Catholicism in the narrative identities of Mexicans and Chicanos on the U.S.-Mexico border.* Paper presented at the annual meeting of the American Sociological Association, Washington, DC.

Wallerstein, N. (1992). Powerlessness, empowerment, and health: Implications for health promotion programs. *American Journal of Health Promotion, 6,* 197-205.

Wallerstein, N., & Bernstein, E. (1988). Empowerment education: Freire's ideas adapted to health education. *Health Education Quarterly, 15,* 379-394.

Zimmerman, M. (1995). Psychological empowerment: Issues and illustrations. *American Journal of Community Psychology, 23,* 581-599.

Zimmerman, M. (in press). Empowerment theory: Psychological, organizational, and community levels of analysis. In J. Rappaport & E. Seidman (Eds.), *The handbook of community psychology.* New York: Plenum.

Zimmerman, M., Janz, N., & Wren, P. (1995). Factors influencing the success of AIDS prevention efforts. In N. Freudenberg & M. Zimmerman (Eds.), *AIDS prevention in the community: Lessons from the first decade.* Washington, DC: American Public Health Association.

Zimmerman, M., Ramirez-Valles, J., Suarez, E., De la Rosa, G., & Castro, M. (1997). An HIV/AIDS prevention project for Mexican homosexual men: An empowering approach. *Health Education and Behavior, 24,* 177-190.

Chapter 8

EASY ACCESS TO CONTRACEPTIVES AMONG FEMALE ADOLESCENTS IN A U.S.-MEXICO BORDER CITY

ELLEN M. PARIETTI
JOÃO B. FERREIRA-PINTO
THERESA BYRD

Access to pharmaceuticals without medical supervision is of concern to health care providers because of patient risk factors, drug interactions, and lack of patient follow-up. This access is of special concern in areas along the U.S.-Mexico border where Mexican pharmacies provide a wide range of prescription pharmaceuticals over the counter. This chapter addresses the use of Mexican pharmacies by young adults living in El Paso, Texas, for the purchase of contraceptives and other pharmaceuticals.

According to the most recent census data (U.S. Bureau of the Census, 1990), 69% of the population of El Paso is of Mexican descent. Research has shown that Mexican Americans seek health care less often than white and black non-Hispanics, Puerto Ricans, and other Hispanics (Estrada, Treviño, & Ray, 1990) and that they underuse preventive services such as routine medical checkups, dental and eye examinations, prenatal care, and family planning (Solis, Marks, Garcia, & Shelton, 1990). Compared to the general population, Hispanics in the United States are less likely to have health insurance and a routine place for health care. This reflects their low levels of income, low levels of formal education, and low levels of acculturation to American society, as well as their lack of knowledge of available resources and having jobs without insurance benefits. Hispanics without health insurance receive half as much medical care as those with health insurance, obtaining fewer physician services and waiting longer between and during physician visits (Solis et al., 1990). Many people living on the U.S.-Mexico border not only buy medications from but also seek health care advice from Mexican pharmacies.

Background

The city of El Paso is a metropolitan center of 503,000 people located in southwest Texas directly on the Mexican border (U.S. Bureau of the Census, 1990). Ciudad Juárez is El Paso's sister city; their downtowns are situated directly across from each other and are separated by only a few blocks. A bridge links the two downtowns, and U.S. residents can cross easily into Ciudad Juárez by car or on foot. Residents of El Paso and Juárez cross back and forth between the two cities, and businesses on both sides of the border are dependent on this behavior. Many El Pasoans are former residents of Juárez or have family and friends that they visit there often. City officials have recognized the interconnectedness of the two cities for years, and issues such as infectious disease, crime, and pollution are considered to affect the commingled population rather than the two distinct ones. The health departments, universities, emergency services, police, and fire departments of both cities collaborate with each other to a large degree.

Just as Juárez residents take advantage of lower prices and perceived better quality of products in the United States, many U.S. residents take advantage of lower prices and lax enforcement of laws regulating Mexican pharmacies. On the Mexican side of the border, though the practice is technically illegal, one can obtain pharmaceuticals without a prescription at a fraction of their U.S. cost. In a pamphlet made available for U.S. visitors to Juárez by the U.S. Customs Service (1992), it is stated that one must have a prescription or written statement from a U.S. physician that the medicine is being used under a doctor's direction and is necessary for one's physical well-being before prescription medicines can be brought across the border. However, this rule is not vigorously enforced. When questioned about the feasibility of the enforcement of this law, a customs official stated that they are lenient in its enforcement, provided that only personal quantities are being imported (R. Vasquez, personal communication, 1994).

One class of medication that women can obtain in Mexico without a doctor's prescription is contraceptives. Both pills and injectable contraceptives can be purchased in Mexico at a fraction of the U.S. cost. A month's cycle of birth control pills can be bought in Juárez pharmacies for between $1 and $3 U.S. A Depo-Provera injection, which provides contraception for 3 months, can be bought for $2 U.S. In comparison, in the United States, pills prescribed by a private physician average $20 U.S. per month. Although in El Paso, birth control pills can be obtained in agencies such as Planned Parenthood on a sliding-scale basis, a Pap smear test must also be conducted and paid for at the time the pills are dispensed. The lowest price for a Pap smear in a public health clinic in El Paso is $20. Depo-Provera costs $46 U.S. in a private physician's office and $35 U.S. at both Planned Parenthood and the University of Texas at El Paso's (UTEP) student health clinic. The required Pap smear and pelvic exam plus the injection would cost $131 U.S. in a private physician's office and $83 U.S. at UTEP (Parietti, 1995).

Because a prescription for birth control pills or injectable contraceptives is not legally required for their purchase in Mexico, women do not have to incur the cost and inconvenience of a gynecological exam, which is required before obtaining contraceptives in the United States. An issue for teenagers is the fact that many doctors and some clinics in the United States still require parental consent for patients below the age of 18 before prescribing a birth control method. This combination of factors provides enough incentive for young women simply to cross the border and obtain over-the-counter contraceptives in Mexico.

Previous Studies

Limited research has examined the utilization of health services in Mexico by U.S. residents. Several factors have been identified as affecting the utilization of Mexican pharmacies. First, Mexican drug prices are a fraction of those charged in U.S. pharmacies (Chavez, Cornelius, & Jones, 1985; Hilts, 1992); second, many recent Mexican immigrants lack access to affordable health care (Hilts, 1992; Myerson, 1994); and third, many express a cultural preference for Mexican therapies, such as vitamins and rehydration solutions administered by injection (Casner & Guerra, 1992;

Parietti, 1995). Preference for Mexican brands sold in individual doses has also been cited. The price differential can be substantial; a box of Tylenol cold medicine costs $4 U.S. in El Paso, whereas a Tabcin tablet, a similar medication, costs only 15 U.S. cents in Mexico (Parietti, 1995).

Only one study was found in the literature that addressed the phenomenon of crossing the U.S.-Mexico border to seek contraceptives in Mexican pharmacies (Smith, Warren, & Garcia-Nuñez, 1983). This study revealed that 9% of Mexican Americans surveyed along the border stated that they traveled across the border into Mexico to get hormonal contraceptive medications. Informal interviews by one of us (Parietti) revealed that many non-Hispanic women also obtain hormonal contraceptives in Juárez.

Description of the Problem

Selling contraceptives over the counter, with proper medical supervision, can be a positive, cost-effective way of ensuring access to birth control for women. However, before hormonal contraceptives are prescribed, a woman should be assessed for health conditions that might contraindicate their use. Information about possible side effects should also be provided. On the basis of both direct observation and testimony given by El Paso women, the above-mentioned type of counseling about risks does not take place in Mexican pharmacies. This can create a series of problems for the women self-medicating without medical supervision. It is important to know to what extent young women are obtaining hormonal methods of birth control without receiving any screening services or information or are using medication that requires a prescription in the United States without medical supervision. In particular, women need to be screened for hypertension, blood clots, and migraines because these are associated with an increased risk of cerebrovascular disorders such as stroke. In addition, because hormonal methods of birth control will rapidly accelerate the growth of cervical cancer, and because sexual activity puts women at greater risk for cervical cancer, Pap smears should be obtained to screen for evidence of this disease.

Risks of Unregulated Medication

The use of hormone-based medications without medical supervision potentially puts the health of women at a great risk. In the United States, to avoid complications and to decrease the incidence of dangerous side effects, women are screened for a variety of conditions before being prescribed hormonal contraception. Most of these conditions are associated with the risk of heart disease or stroke. For instance, significant increase in blood pressure has been associated with both the estrogen and the progestin in birth control pills. Women should have their blood pressure checked before starting hormonal contraceptives and then should continue to monitor it. If the blood pressure rises to over 90 mm Hg, oral contraceptives should be discontinued or changed to a lower dose. Other conditions that would contraindicate the use of oral contraceptives are diabetes mellitus, gestational diabetes (both of which are very common in the Mexican population), thrombophlebitis, heart disease or a history thereof, migraine headaches, and continued smoking (Hatcher et al., 1994). A physician or a conscientious pharmacist should inquire about these conditions before prescribing birth control pills.

Depo-Provera is an injectable contraceptive gaining popularity in the United States because it is convenient and long lasting; its dosage is administered only once every 3 months. There are two contraindications for Depo-Provera use: existing undetected pregnancy and unexplained abnormal vaginal bleeding. Women should have pregnancy tests done before injections are started because the drug can cause birth defects. Also, any unexplained vaginal bleeding should be diagnosed by a clinician before Depo-Provera injections are prescribed (Hatcher et al., 1994). Depo-Provera usually leads to irregular menses and increased days of light bleeding or spotting and so may mask an underlying problem such as pelvic inflammatory disease, cancer of the reproductive tract, or pregnancy, which may have similar symptoms.

During informal preliminary interviews, a number of El Paso women reported purchases of contraceptive pills and injections in Mexican pharmacies. Perlutal is the brand name of the drug that El Paso women most reported purchasing. It is an injectable contraceptive that is administered once a month. Not available in the United States, Perlutal was identified by the Department of Health Services in California (State of California, 1992) as one of several "potentially unsafe and illegal drug products being sold within the Hispanic communities." Perlutal is also one of a number of drugs from Mexico being sold in flea markets in southern California. The Food and Drug Branch could not correct the problem by confiscating the drugs because the sellers and users did not understand the potential dangers of these products and described the raids in "flea markets" and *botánicas* (herbal stores) as discrimination against Mexican Americans. To educate all Californians about the dangers of these products when used without medical supervision, the Pharmaceutical Manufacturers Association (PMA) was asked for assistance in designing and financing an effective statewide campaign because many member companies of the PMA manufacture and sell within Mexico many of the drug products being sold illegally in California. The product of this collaboration between the PMA and the state of California is the manual *Potentially Dangerous Imported Spanish Labeled Prescription Drug Products,* prepared by the State of California Department of Health Services Food and Drug Branch (1992). Information on Perlutal published in this manual states: "Adverse effects: menstrual irregularities and breakthrough bleeding, hormonal imbalance, hypertension, cancerous and non-cancerous liver tumors. Public health concerns: may cause cancer; may cause birth defects if used while pregnant. For intramuscular injection only. Safe administration of injectable drugs requires training" (State of California, 1992).

Casner, an El Paso physician, called the actions of these women a unique United States-Mexico border phenomenon: that is, U.S. residents crossing the border into Mexico to take advantage of the different regulations surrounding pharmaceuticals (Casner & Guerra, 1992). Because Mexican pharmacies sell drugs not approved for sale in the United States and at a lower price, border health practitioners are worried about the potential harm of unregulated self-medication and complications resulting from unsupervised consumption of these medications.

Mexican pharmacists and other pharmacy employees without formal training are accustomed to recommending drugs for treatments for which they have not been approved by the Food and Drug Administration (FDA) in the United States, such as steroids for the treatment of arthritis and asthma. This particular use of steroids can cause serious long-term health effects. Casner and Guerra (1992) also stated that physicians should be aware that a patient's self-medication could confuse his or her diagnosis. A toxicologist at El Paso's Thomason Hospital says that he frequently treats patients who have gotten sick from medication they bought over the counter in Juárez without first consulting a doctor. A common problem is children whose parents have given them diarrhea medication containing sedatives. Because doctors often depend on a child's level of activity to assist in determining how sick a child is, tests must be run to see if the child has a serious illness or is simply reacting to a medication (Negron, 1992).

Another important public health concern is the potential development of drug-resistant strains of bacteria resulting from indiscriminate antibiotic use that could affect both countries' populations (Casner, 1984; Rubin,

SeGatt, & Audette, 1990). In Juárez, antibiotics are available without prescription, package insert information is poor, and there is no national antibiotic use program. Antibiotics are used liberally and often inappropriately. When an antibiotic becomes widely prescribed by physicians, the general public concludes that it is useful for all types of infections, and the process of automedication begins. Rodriguez-Noriega, Morfin-Otero, and Esparza-Ahumada (1993) suggested that all antimicrobials should be available only by prescription, pertinent information should be included in a package insert, and all countries should implement a comprehensive antibiotic usage program to control bacterial resistance and maintain the effectiveness of antibiotics.

There has been recent concern regarding the increase in drug-resistant illnesses (particularly tuberculosis) and the role that indiscriminate or inappropriate medication may play in this. One case in point is a commercial suspension containing Rifampin (used to treat tuberculosis) that is manufactured in Mexico and has been recommended by many Mexican pharmacies for children with coughs (Gellert & Pyle, 1994).

Another danger in the use of medications without medical supervision involves possible drug interactions that can occur when taking more than one drug. *Polypharmacy* is the term for the concomitant use of multiple medications. Persons who obtain medicines from unsupervised or multiple sources run the risk of potentially serious adverse effects resulting from the interaction of multiple medications. In the United States, pharmacists commonly track their clients' medications and alert doctors of any possible interactions. This type of safeguard is not available to those who use Mexican pharmacies (R. Alvord, personal communication, April 10, 1995).

Many drugs sold in Mexican pharmacies without a prescription are in injectable form, and safe administration of these medications can be an issue. Receiving injections from untrained persons without confirming the sterility of the needle, syringe, and medication puts the purchaser at risk for HIV, hepatitis B, and other infections. Other potential dangers from unqualified people injecting medicine include bleeding, nerve damage, and allergic reactions (R. Alvord, personal communication, April 10, 1995). For example, children have been admitted to El Paso's Thomason Hospital with a series of symptoms resulting from an injectable antibiotic administrated incorrectly by their mothers (Casner, 1984). Because El Paso women have said that Mexican American women have become accustomed to sharing needles freely when administering antibiotics and vitamins, AIDS educators in the area, such as those who attended the April 1994 Conferencia de la Mujer Trabajadora Agricola Fronteriza Contra el Sida, are also stressing the importance of not sharing needles and using only sterile needles when injecting any drugs.

Although health care providers along the border see use of Mexican pharmacies as a potentially dangerous situation, they also understand that for low-income U.S. residents, access to the Mexican pharmacies may be the only way for them to afford the health care they need.

Purpose

The purpose of this research was to describe the extent of use of Mexican pharmacies for the contraceptive medication needs of young adults living in El Paso. In addition, this study was designed to gather information about the use of Mexican pharmacies for the over-the-counter purchase of other medications that cannot be obtained in the United States without a prescription.

Methodology

In this study, a descriptive methodology was used to examine the practices of young men and women in El Paso regarding their use of Mexican pharmacies for contraceptive medication and other pharmaceutical needs. Preliminary informal interviews were conducted with El Paso residents who admitted to the use of Mexican pharmacies. These interviews ($n = 10$) revealed a variety of reasons for buying pharmaceuticals in Mexico, but the lower cost of drugs was mentioned most often. Subjects also cited the lack of need for a prescription, which eliminates the cost of a doctor's appointment (and possibly the need to take off from work to see the doctor), and the lower prices offered in Juárez pharmacies. Other reasons cited were the availability of certain Mexican products not found in the United States and a preference for the type of therapies found in Mexico, especially injectables.

Additional preliminary interviews were conducted with nine El Paso women: five UTEP students and four working women. Three of the four working women stated that they had purchased an injectable contraceptive in Juárez. Three of the students stated that many of their friends had purchased contraceptives in Mexican pharmacies and that during high school it was common for girls to purchase contraceptives in Mexico. Two of the students reported having purchased diet pills in Mexico and said that this was a common practice.

Unsuccessful attempts were made to collect information from pharmacists in Juárez during the purchase of contraceptives. The availability of birth control pills and injections was discussed with pharmacy employees, and advice was sought about which contraceptive to take. If no counsel was offered, the request was made for the pharmacist in charge to answer the questions regarding contraindications or side effects. These attempts were unsuccessful because the pharmacists, although polite, never answered the questions posed. In addition, the purchase of diet pills and other medications was discussed with employees at the counter in the pharmacies visited. All interviews in Mexican pharmacies were conducted in Spanish. The methodology employed in the pharmacies was ethnographic observation in a public situation and did not include access to confidential information or invasion of privacy.

To learn more about the use of over-the-counter contraceptives by El Paso youth, a survey of freshman female and male college students attending the local university and community college was conducted. In addition to demographic questions, the survey asked specific questions about sexual practices, the use of birth control, the purchase of contraceptives, screening for cervical cancer, smoking, health conditions, and the purchases of diuretics and other medication in Juárez pharmacies.

Students' Survey

The survey instrument was approved by the human subjects review committee. Students were informed that participation was totally voluntary and that they were free to decline. The survey was anonymous; no names or signatures were used. It was therefore explained that the act of filling out the survey indicated consent, and those that declined turned in a blank form with a declination indicated on top, such as "I decline." The survey sample consisted of 160 male and 201 female college students enrolled in introductory psychology classes at UTEP. The course is a requirement for psychology majors and is popular among all students. The freshman-level psychology classes' age and ethnic profile is representative of the entire student body of UTEP. Sixty-nine percent of undergraduate psychology majors are Hispanic (Ronco, Passmore, & Monteros, 1994). The undergraduate student body at UTEP is 66% Hispanic, and 88% are El Paso residents (Ronco et al., 1994). Eighty-four students from El Paso Community College (EPCC) were also surveyed. Tuition at EPCC is significantly lower than at UTEP, thereby allowing students with fewer financial resources to enroll in classes. Inclusion of this population made the sample more representative of young El Paso men and women on the whole. The students surveyed at EPCC were also enrolled in freshman-level psychology classes. The EPCC sample consisted of 30 men and 54 women, bringing the total survey sample to 445 students (190 men and 255 women).

Survey Results

As shown in Table 8.1, the mean age for the women in this survey was 21.6 years and for the men was 22.1 years. Most of the students identified their ethnic backgrounds as Hispanic (80.4% of the men and 78.5% of the women), with non-Hispanic white being the second-largest group (12.2% of the men and 15.6% of the women). There was a small representation of African Americans (eight men and six women), and "other" (six men and nine women), who were mainly Asian.

Sexual Practices

In responses to the question "Have you ever engaged in sexual intercourse?" more than three fourths of the men and two thirds of the women responded affirmatively. This subgroup will be referred to as "sexually experienced" in the text. Those who had engaged in sexual intercourse were asked whether they had done so in the last 30 days. Of the sexually experienced participants, more than half the men and more than two thirds of the women indicated that they had done so in the last 30 days. This subpopulation will be referred to from here on as "sexually active."

Use of Birth Control

Table 8.2 lists all the birth control methods ever used by sexually experienced participants and their partners (current and past). Experience with condoms appears to be very widespread among both sexes, with 81% of men and 80% of women reporting their use. Use of injectable contraceptives, diaphragms, Norplant, and intrauterine devices are low among

TABLE 8.1 Age Distribution and Ethnic Background

	Males	n	Females	n
Age				
17-18	17.3%	33	29.5%	78
19-20	44.2%	85	41.6%	106
21-24	22.6%	42	12.6%	32
>24	15.9%	30	16.3%	44
Mean age	22.1 $SD = 7.04$		21.6 $SD = 6.63$	
Ethnic background				
White non-Hispanic	12.2%	23	15.6%	40
Hispanic	80.4%	152	78.5%	201
African American	4.2%	8	2.3%	6
Other	3.2%	6	3.5%	9

both men's sexual partners and women. There are marked differences between the sexes on the reported use of certain birth control methods. Though only 13.1% of men reported that their partners had used birth control pills, 46.7% of women reported having done so. Also, only 2% of the men stated that their partners had used natural family planning, whereas 18.6% of the women reported having used this method. Thirty percent of women reported that their sexual partners had used withdrawal as a method of birth control, and only 18.2% of the men surveyed reported having used this method themselves.

Purchase of Contraceptive Medication in Mexican Pharmacies

In response to the question "Have you ever obtained birth control pills or injectable contraceptives such as Depo Provera from pharmacies in Mexico?" 92% of the women responded negatively. Of those who said they had obtained birth control in Mexico ($n = 12$), 11 had purchased oral contraceptives, and 1 had purchased Depo Provera.

TABLE 8.2 Birth Control Methods Ever Used by Sexually Experienced
            Participants or Their Partners

	Men	*n*	*Women*	*n*
Condoms	81%	136	80%	91
Oral contraceptives	13.1%	20	46.7%	77
Injections	3.5%	4	7.9%	11
Diaphragm	3.2%	5	2.5%	4
Norplant	2.0%	1	2.5%	4
Withdrawal	18.2%	28	30%	49
IUD	2.0%	1	7.7%	13
Natural family planning	2.0%	1	18.6%	30

Screening for Cervical Cancer

Of the 12 women who had purchased birth control pills or injectable contraceptives in Mexico, 7 indicated that they had *not* received regular Pap smears during that time, and 5 reported that they had received Pap smears. Of the 12 women purchasing contraceptive medication in Juárez, 2 (16.7%) had received information regarding warnings of possible side effects, and 10 (83.3%) had not.

*Male Responses About
Female Friends' Behaviors*

Males were asked in the survey, "Have you been aware of friends or partners obtaining birth control pills or injectable contraceptives in Mexico?" Twenty-one percent ($n = 40$) reported that they had and 78.4% ($n = 145$) that they had not. Of those who responded affirmatively, 75% indicated that birth control pills were being purchased, and the remainder indicated the purchase of injectable contraceptives. When asked if these women had been under the care of a gynecologist at the time of the contraceptive use, 18.4% of the men indicated that the women had not been under the care of a gynecologist, 5.8% said that they had been, and 65.8% said that they did not know. When asked if these women had experienced any side effects from the pills or injections, 25.6% of the men indicated that the women had not, 7.7% said that they had, and 66.7% did not know.

Smoking and Use of Oral Contraceptives

In addition to being asked about the methods of birth control that they used, sexually experienced women were asked about certain health conditions that could constitute contraindications against certain hormonal methods of birth control. First, women were asked if they smoked. Twenty-two percent responded affirmatively. Of the smokers, 75% reported smoking under a pack per week.

Health Conditions Constituting Risk Factors
for Contraceptive Medicines

Women were asked if they had experienced blood clots of any kind, heart disease or a family history of it, tumors or a family history of them, migraines, diabetes, high blood pressure, severe abdominal pain, severe chest pain, headaches with dizziness, vision problems, or severe leg pain. Participants were to check all responses that applied. Some of the more significant findings included the prevalence of migraines; 19% of all women surveyed reported suffering from migraines. Among the women using birth control pills (which are contraindicated for women who suffer migraines), those obtaining the pills in Mexico had a higher prevalence of migraines (75%) than those who were obtaining them in the United States and, as required, had to be under the care of a physician (18.8%).

Diuretics/Weight Control

Eighteen (7.7%) of the women sampled responded that they had purchased diuretics or other weight control drugs. Men were asked if their friends/sexual partners had purchased medicine in Mexico to lose weight or reduce water retention. Thirty-six percent said no, 21% said yes, and 43% said they were not sure.

Other Medications Purchased
in Mexican Pharmacies

Forty-four percent of the men and 55% of the women reported that they did use Mexican pharmacies for the purchase of medications, as shown in Table 8.3.

Those reporting having done so were then asked what types of medicines they bought in the pharmacies: medication prescribed by the doctor,

TABLE 8.3 Distribution of Survey Participants Who Report Purchasing
Medicine in Mexican Pharmacies

	Men	n	Women	n
Yes	44.4%	79	55.1%	135
No	55.6%	98	44.9%	110

medication prescribed without a prescription, medicine suggested by the pharmacist on inquiry about a specific problem/ailment, or over-the-counter medicine. Participants were asked to mark all responses that applied. Three percent of the women and 36.7% of the men who used medicines purchased in Mexico said that they had purchased medicines prescribed them by their doctor. The most commonly purchased were antibiotics and allergy medicines. Sixty percent of the men and 63.4% of the women surveyed said that they bought medications without a doctor's prescription in Mexican pharmacies. The majority of these purchases were antibiotics, but purchases also included a wide variety of other medications, such as bronchiodilators, muscle relaxants, allergy medicines, diuretics, estrogen, and cold and flu medications. Thirty-three percent of women and 19% of men reported buying medicine suggested to them by the pharmacist on inquiry about a specific problem/ailment.

When a chi-square test was used to examine the association between ethnicity and a number of behaviors related to drug purchase in Mexican pharmacies, the only statistically significant result was between ethnicity and the purchase of medications other than contraceptives and diuretics (χ = 13.28, p = .016). Women of Hispanic descent were more likely to use Juárez pharmacies for the purchase of medicines *other* than contraceptive medication or diuretics.

Interviews in Juárez Pharmacies

During visits to the pharmacies, one of us (Parietti) was attended to by pharmacy employees—in all but three cases, by young women employees. In every instance, the *farmacia* employees failed to offer any advice on possible side effects or drug interactions, even though they were informed that no hormonal birth control had ever been used before by the customer.

Never was the pharmacist present in a supervisory fashion. In three instances, a pharmacist was summoned to answer questions regarding side effects and counterindications for injections and birth control pills. On two of these occasions, the pharmacists were not very attentive and never answered questions before leaving to take care of other things. In one case, when it was first explained to the attendant that no birth control pills or injections had ever been used, the attendant listed the options available and suggested that perhaps the advice of a doctor should be sought first.

When asked if many El Paso residents came to buy medicine in the Mexican pharmacies, all *farmacia* employees responded affirmatively. "Especially on weekends," volunteered a few. The employees reported that antibiotics were bought most frequently, but they stated that they sell all kinds of medications, such as allergy medicines and ulcer medication. When asked, "Do many women come to buy birth control pills and injections here?" all answered yes. "What are these women like?" "Like you," one woman said, referring to one of us (Parietti), a young white non-Hispanic female. Two pharmacies stated that they sold a lot of Perlutal to U.S. residents, and the other five pharmacies stated that for the most part people came from El Paso to buy birth control pills (all specifying Ortho-Novum brand pills) and did not tend to buy the injections (Perlutal and Depo-Provera). The UTEP/EPCC students surveyed seemed to reflect this: 90% of the El Paso students buying hormonal methods of birth control in Juárez were buying birth control pills.

While we discussed the option of injectable contraception, we explored the issue of the injection itself. Both Depo-Provera and Perlutal are sold in an ampoule. When asked, "Who would inject me?" the most common response was, "Many people know how to inject." Only one of the pharmacies offered the service of injection. A needle can be purchased for the equivalent of 50 U.S. cents, and the service of injecting the medication would cost another $1 U.S. When asked about the technical preparation required to give injections, the employee answered that all the staff had attended instruction on giving injections. In other interviews with women who had purchased injectable birth control in Juárez, it was reported that there are women who know how to inject and will administer injections in their homes for you.

Inquiries were also made into the sale of diet pills. Informal interviews indicated that it was common for women to purchase pills designed to help reduce fluid retention and/or lose weight. When asked if it was common for U.S. residents to come looking for such medications, all *farmacia* employees answered yes.

Discussion

The college student survey revealed that 8% (n = 12) of sexually experienced women obtained contraceptive pills or injections in Mexican pharmacies and that 22% (n = 40) of the male students had friends or partners who were doing so. The difference in the data between men's and women's reported use of Mexican pharmacies as a contraceptive source suggests that some of the male students may have partners who are not their school peers and that those women may be different because of age or income. The results of the informal preliminary interviews led us to believe that the number of women buying hormonal contraceptives in Juárez would be higher, but even 8% of a student population engaging in this practice is of significant concern to health authorities. Women informants in the preliminary informal interviews who reported the purchase of oral or injection contraceptives in Mexico either were working or had been working in the past few years and were roughly 4 to 6 years older on average than the survey participants. Employment status and age could account for their differences in using Mexican pharmacies as contraceptive sources. Students qualify for special school health care services at reduced prices and may be using these services for birth control. Women who were informally interviewed, although working, may have had poor insurance coverage or no insurance at all, encouraging their use of Juárez pharmacies for health care services, including birth control.

The practice of obtaining contraceptive medication without medical supervision can be dangerous and poses risks to women with preexisting conditions and certain high-risk behaviors. These conditions include migraine headaches, hypertension, blood clots, heart problems, and smoking. They are related to an increased risk of strokes and emboli (clots) associated with the use of contraceptive medication. Because 75% (n = 6) of the survey participants who obtained birth control pills in Mexican pharmacies reported experiencing migraine headaches and 33% (n = 4) were smokers, the lack of medical supervision and counseling is of particular concern.

Unsupervised use of these prescription medications raises other concerns. Self-medication confuses the diagnosis of physicians when patients eventually do seek medical attention from professionals. Patients may suffer drug interactions from taking more than one medication without receiving counsel. Antibiotics should be used only in cases of a laboratory-confirmed microbial infection that is known to be susceptible to the drug. Patients should be advised that the full course of treatment must be completed if antibiotic efficacy is to be obtained. This will help avoid the production of antibiotic-resistant strains of bacteria. Of the seven medicines most commonly purchased by respondents, five were listed in the manual *Potentially Dangerous Imported Spanish Labeled Prescription Drug Products* (State of California, 1992). Of the medications that respondents reported purchasing in Mexican pharmacies, 12 were listed as potentially dangerous, some due to side effects, others for the risks they pose to pregnant women and children, and others because they are unapproved for use in the United States.

Both injectable contraceptives, Depo-Provera (available in the United States) and Perlutal (available in Mexico but not in the United States), cause birth defects if administered to pregnant women. With neither medical supervision nor counsel given on purchase, a woman might take the medication before realizing she was pregnant.

One third of the women who report purchasing hormonal methods of birth control in this study also report using Mexican pharmacies for the purchase of antibiotics. Given that no advice or warnings are given with the sale of medications, there is concern that some drug interactions may take place, affecting the efficacy of birth control pills.

Conclusions

Fifty-five percent of the women ($n = 135$) and 44% of the men ($n = 79$) surveyed reported using Mexican pharmacies for the purchase of medications, including those requiring a prescription in the United States. These numbers reflect a prevalence of use of Mexican pharmacies far above that which had been expected for a young, presumably healthy population. Because there are other populations in El Paso with a higher dependence on medications, such as the sick and elderly, the prevalence of this behavior in El Paso is expected to be higher than that found in this study. There are many retired people in El Paso, some of whom require several medications. Many of them rely on Mexican pharmacies to cut costs and are at risk for negative drug reactions associated with polypharmacy. Children also are at particular risk when taking medications without medical supervision. Mothers use Mexican pharmacies to medicate their children either because they feel confident about treating their child's illnesses after years of visiting pediatricians or because they cannot afford the expense involved in taking their children to a doctor. Special caution should be exercised because many adult medicines are dangerous when administered to children. Medication dosage is dependent on the weight of the child, and correct administration requires some calculation and transformations to and from the metric system. Finally, children have an increased incidence of allergic reactions to medications and should be watched closely for signs of such a reaction.

The fact that large numbers of people feel the need to seek pharmaceuticals in Mexico calls for a reexamination of our health care system in the United States. El Paso and other towns along the Mexican border are unique in that their populations have access to alternative solutions to their health care needs. Others in cities far from the Mexican border have responded to this desire for access to pharmaceuticals without prescriptions by searching for alternative buying options. For instance, vendors in southern California are selling medicine originally purchased in Mexico at flea markets. In New York City, an investigative reporter documented the sale of antibiotics without prescription in four Brooklyn pharmacies (Trotter, 1995).

As long as there exists an opportunity for significant savings by purchasing medications in Mexico, people will continue to use Mexican pharmacies for their needs. The availability of medication at such reduced prices makes it possible for many uninsured people to treat medical conditions. It is our opinion that the danger presented by Mexican pharmacies and their custom of selling over-the-counter medications would be minimized if customers and pharmacy employees were more aware of the side effects of commonly acquired medicines, contraindications, and drug interactions of certain medications so that customers would be better protected.

Due to the serious nature of some of the potential side effects and interactions of these medications, a more extensive and formal investigation of the use of Mexican pharmacies by El Paso residents should be undertaken. A stratified sample more representative of the entire El Paso population should be surveyed, including all age groups and socioeconomic levels, to explore their use of Mexican pharmacies. Information on the frequency with which they use them, the medications purchased, the extent of doctor supervision, and the reasons for going to Mexico for these services should be explored. Special populations, such as the elderly and women with young children, for which there is anecdotal evidence of their use of Mexican pharmacies but for which there are no substantive data should be also be included. In addition, studies might be conducted in which El Paso residents making medication purchases in Mexican pharmacies would be observed and interviewed. It should be determined what they are buying as well as the factors that influence their decision to shop in Mexican pharmacies.

The purchase of prescription medications over the counter is a common occurrence that is unique to the U.S.-Mexico border area. Both the benefits and the dangers are real. Programs to educate the public about proper use of prescription drugs and their possible side effects are a first step that should be taken to avoid public health problems. Enforcement of policies already in place to prevent the misuse of prescription drugs, although difficult, should be a priority. Finally, the U.S. health care and drug manufacturing systems should be reformed to allow for the availability of affordable health care for all.

References

Casner, P. R. (1984). Antibiotics over the counter and across the border. *Annals of Internal Medicine, 100,* 462-463.

Casner, P. R., & Guerra, L. G. (1992). Purchasing prescription medication in Mexico without a prescription: The experience at the border. *Western Journal of Medicine, 156,* 512-516.

Chavez, L. R., Cornelius, W. A., & Jones, O. W. (1985). Mexican immigrants and the utilization of U.S. health care services: The case of San Diego. *Western Journal of Medicine, 21,* 93-102.

Estrada, A. L., Treviño, F. M., & Ray, L. A. (1990). Health care utilization barriers among Mexican Americans: Evidence from HHANES 1982-84. *American Journal of Public Health, 80*(Suppl.), 27-31.

Gellert, G. A., & Pyle, N. G. (1994). Pharmacy practice and antibiotic-resistant tuberculosis along the U.S.-Mexican border. *Journal of the American Medical Association, 271,* 1577-1578.

Hatcher, R., Guest, F., Stewart, F., Stewart, G., Trussell, J., Bowen, S. C., & Cates, W. (1994). *Contraceptive technology* (16th Rev. ed.). New York: Irvington.

Hilts, P. (1992, November 22). Quality and low cost of medical care lure Americans to Mexican doctors. *New York Times,* p. 11.

Myerson, A. (1994, September 29). Jeans makers flourish on border. *New York Times,* p. C1.

Negron, S. (1992, May 25). Juarez medicine called a trade-off. *El Paso Times,* p. B1.

Parietti, E. (1995). *Young women's use of Mexican pharmacies as a contraceptive provider.* Unpublished master's thesis, University of Texas at Houston Health Science Center, El Paso.

Rodriguez-Noriega, E., Morfin-Otero, R., & Esparza-Ahumada, S. (1993). The use of quinolones in developing countries. *Drugs, 45*(Suppl. 3), 42-45.

Ronco, S., Passmore, B., & Monteros, B. (1994). *The University of Texas at El Paso fact book 1993-94.* El Paso: University of Texas at El Paso, Office of Institutional Studies.

Rubin, B. K., SeGatt, D. F., & Audette, R. J. (1990). The Mexican asthma cure: Systematic steroids for gullible gringos. *Chest, 97,* 959-961.

Smith, J. C., Warren, C. W., & Garcia-Nuñez, J. (1983). *The U.S.-Mexico border: Contraceptive use and maternal health care in perspective, 1979*. El Paso, TX: United States-Mexico Border Health Association.

Solis, J. M., Marks, G., Garcia, M., & Shelton, D. (1990). Acculturation, access to care, and use of preventive services by Hispanics: Findings from HHANES 1982-84. *American Journal of Public Health, 80*(Suppl.), 11-19.

State of California, Department of Health Services, Food and Drug Branch. (1992). *Potentially dangerous imported Spanish labeled prescription drug products (Version 1.0)*. Unpublished document.

Trotter, E. (1995, January 3). Rx for disaster: Not what the doc ordered. *New York Post,* p. 4.

U.S. Bureau of the Census. (1990). *Census of population and housing*. Washington, DC: Government Printing Office.

U.S. Customs Service. (1992). *Know before you go: Customs hints for returning residents* (Pub. No. 512). Washington, DC: Department of the Treasury.

Part 3

~~~

Models for Health Promotion
in the Border Region

A great benefit of the research that has been conducted in public health is not only the insight that has been gained about people's health behaviors but also the dissemination of information regarding successful practices and models that can be replicated in other contexts and with other populations. Whether one's ideas actually work in practice is ultimately the greatest test of the theory. This section offers three such models that in many ways are unique to the border environment but that could, no doubt, be replicated in part, if not entirely, in other locations with similar demographics.

The three models proposed in this section offer different approaches to health promotion based on three levels of analysis: individual, structural, and programmatic. Although these levels of analysis are not mutually exclusive, the authors focus on one particular element rather than the other two. In each case, the authors identify the strengths and weaknesses of each model and the obstacles that are likely to be encountered when adopting these approaches. The models proposed are particularly sensitive to the populations they serve in terms of differences in gender, language proficiency, and literacy levels and to the characteristics of the border environment.

Chapter 9

✧

BOUNDARY SPANNERS

Las Promotoras *in the Borderlands*

LEIGH ARDEN FORD
MICHAEL D. BARNES
ROBBIN D. CRABTREE
JO FAIRBANKS

The trend toward community-based health workers is favorably acknowledged by health and public health professionals as essential for the ever-changing arena of health care in rural and urban areas along the U.S.-Mexico border and beyond. In this chapter, we discuss community health worker (CHW) or *promotora* ("promoter") projects along the southwestern border of the United States, with particular attention to the rural areas of southern New Mexico and west Texas. At minimum, the *promotoras* provide a much-needed link to health care resources for community members. However, in most cases, they also provide other functions vital to the health, well-being, and general development of their communities.

In our view, the unifying and defining principle of all the role enactments of the *promotora* is *boundary spanning*. These CHWs cross boundaries of age, gender, education, social class, and culture in their role performance. The traditional boundaries associated with health and human service providers are bridged by CHWs. The definitional boundaries of health and illness in a community are reexamined by community members with the aid of *promotoras*. Finally, the disciplinary and research boundaries of public health and communication paradigms are crossed within an examination of *promotora* programs. The ability to go beyond these constraints and to bridge these differences is the great strength and continual challenge of these CHWs.

Our goal in this chapter is to enumerate the multiple roles that *las promotoras* fill within their communities. First, we provide a definition and general description of the CHW model. We then discuss the structure of CHW programs generally and specific characteristics of these programs in the southwestern United States. We also provide a discussion of the training of these community workers, including the necessary components, resources, and strategies of training. We then focus our attention specifically on the constellation of roles enacted by the *promotora* from a public health perspective and from a communication perspective. We conclude with a discussion of the barriers to effective boundary spanning encountered by CHWs as they perform their community activities.

The Challenges of Public Health and Communication in the Borderlands

A 2,000-mile-long stretch of land across the continent defines the border between the United States and Mexico. This physical representation does not and cannot capture the unique and complex blend of social, economic, political, and cultural factors that ultimately constitute the territory known as "the borderlands." Any examination of health status and health care must be understood within this context and within an appreciation of the character of mutual dependence and day-to-day interaction among the peoples of both sides of the border. The problems of mortality and morbidity within the border populations of southern New Mexico and west Texas can be traced to a complex interaction among these multiple factors (Ortega, 1992).

First, this area is largely rural, with a few large cities interspersed. This geographic vastness creates a physical isolation from services and from other community members. This distance limits ready access to information about health-related issues and to the health care delivery source itself. In addition, the residents of border areas generally have a low educational level and economic status. Though some economic opportunities are emerging along the border, generally the developing job market continues to provide relatively low-wage jobs (Ortega, 1992). This reduced economic status and educational attainment of borderland residents create considerable barriers to access to health services, to knowledge about health-related issues, and to the potential to effect change in these systems.

Another factor contributing to the challenges of improving health status in the borderlands is the meeting and melding of multiple cultures. The dominant Hispanic and Anglo cultural traditions and customs, combined with the cultural influences of some Native American tribes, add a richness and diversity to life along the border. These self-same linguistic and cultural beliefs and traditions simultaneously create barriers to effective health care delivery and to effective communication regarding health-related information and specific health practices.

Finally, the very permeability of the border is a challenge to public health and communication practitioners. Currently, the U.S. Census Bureau projects continued growth for the southwestern United States and a decline in population growth in other parts of the country. The region's growth rate is explained by an increasing number of immigrants and by higher birth rates among the population of the Southwest. For example, between 1980 and 1990, New Mexico had a 14% population expansion, and that rate of population increase is expected to continue. Further, in the borderlands, individuals continue to move back and forth between the two countries with some regularity, depending on current economic conditions in the United States and in Mexico. Consequently, the number of persons in need of health and human services in the southwestern United States continues to grow. Meanwhile, already fragmented, underfunded, and underresourced, the existing health and human service system of the area is severely stretched in its efforts to provide services (Ortega, 1992).

Population growth has also led to a sort of urban development that is largely unregulated and that has resulted in the construction of substandard housing. Along the U.S. border, particularly in Texas and southern New Mexico, these rural subdivisions, or *colonias,* often lack electricity, plumbing, sewage disposal systems, and access to clean, potable water. These environmental problems contribute significantly to the overall lower health status of border communities.

In sum, the economic, social, and cultural challenges are great in the borderlands. These challenges must be met if we are to see improved mortality and morbidity rates in the region. Meeting these challenges will require multiple strategies developed and enacted by institutions and by individuals. These strategies include a renewed commitment to the principle of universal access, cross-border governmental cooperation, grassroots organizing for community development, and the development and implementation of alternative strategies for increasing access to health and disease prevention information and for linking individuals to the health and human service infrastructure.

The CHW Model

One strategy that has been developed to address the complexities associated with improving the health status of individuals and with encouraging grassroots community development along the border is the CHW model. This model has been implemented in developing countries and in both rural and urban settings in the United States (Brownstein & Wilson, 1994; Centers for Disease Control and Prevention [CDC], 1994a, 1994b; Walker, 1994). In the following sections, we provide a definition and description of the CHW model. We describe program components and structures and outline training strategies. Again, we focus our specific attention on the model as it is represented in *promotora* projects in southern New Mexico and west Texas.

CHWs: Definition and Program Description

CHWs are "trusted and respected community members who provide informal, community based health-related services" (CDC, 1994a, p. vi) and who establish vital links between health professionals and persons in the community (CDC, 1994a, 1994b). They act to increase the accessibility, acceptability, and appropriateness of available health services (Office of Migrant Health, 1992). In areas where CHWs are serving, they are able to communicate with providers about the needs of community members, provide quality health promotion and disease prevention information to the community, and serve as a critical link between their community and health practitioners to increase use of available preventive health services. They assist residents within the community to obtain available health and human services and provide outreach to those who may not be aware of those services. They become the voice of the community, resonating with true understanding of community needs and issues. CHWs are trusted by and supported by their neighbors and communities to increase the effectiveness of the health care delivery system, reduce preventable morbidity and mortality, and improve the quality of life (Walker, 1994; Woodruff, 1994).

As local, indigenous residents of underserved communities, CHWs are uniquely knowledgeable about their populations' needs. Further, CHWs offer a promising community-based method for affecting hard-to-reach priority populations, specifically minority and low-income populations (Larson, 1992). As respected members of a particular community, CHWs are able to go into the homes of community members and build a link between a family and the assortment of health, social, education, and care resources that are available in the community to meet the family's needs (International Medical Services for Health [INMED], 1993). Thus, CHWs are not trained to substitute for professionals but act as complements to health providers, with a mission to improve health in ways that traditional educators and care providers are not able to provide (Barnes, 1995).

The *promotora* projects of southern New Mexico and west Texas are also defined by the previously described parameters. *Promotoras* come from the area where they work; they are adults, usually women, with a minimum amount of formal education. Within their communities, they are trained to provide support and health-related information to an identified population, usually one not currently accessing the health care or human services network. They are volunteers or paid workers, usually assisting the current system to improve the lives of others through a more equitable distribution of services. *Promotoras* along the border face the special challenges of the borderland described previously. They interact with a population that is poor, geographically isolated, and often suspicious and fearful of the existing health and human services network. However, as members of the community and the culture, they bring to their work the language, cultural understanding, and shared worldview of members of the community in ways that other health providers cannot approximate.[1]

Within the past 5 years, increasing health care costs, limited health care access, and growing priority populations have stimulated interest in CHWs. For example, the U.S. General Accounting Office (1990) identified home visiting by community health advisors as a promising strategy that assists at-risk families in becoming healthier and more self-sufficient, as well as reducing later serious and costly problems. This report also identified low-income, less educated, or teen-headed families as the populations that benefit most from these activities. CHW programs are increasingly winning support for the prospects and outcomes related to preventing problems rather than relying on costly, curative solutions (INMED, 1993).

However, CHW projects should not be viewed as a panacea for current problems in health and human services delivery. CHW projects must have a support structure in place before attempting to reach out to a given population. In the border regions of the United States, that infrastructure can be very fragmented. Improved access to health care is no substitute for adequate nutrition, potable water, and a basic standard of living. The value of CHWs to their communities is significant, but they are not a substitute for access to adequate health and human services. Although their activities are often useful and low in cost, these workers are not the only answer to the crisis in health care for poor, underserved populations.

In addition, CHW programs have potential liabilities. Gottlieb (1985) suggested that social network interactions (such as those of CHWs within their communities) can have negative and positive consequences. For example, well-intentioned help perceived as too demanding or too controlling by the recipient can create a sort of backlash. Further, Steckler, Dawson, Israel, and Eng (1993) pointed out that CHW programs can be expensive and time consuming and can have less-than-adequate recording and reporting practices, questionable data collection procedures, and invalid/unreliable assessment or evaluation instruments. Finally, Steckler et al. (1993) explained that CHW efforts may not address actual causes of the problem(s) or may distract from more basic societal changes that are needed and thus impede the actual progress sought. It is also possible for CHWs to compete against trained professionals, claiming that their more personalized approach is superior.

It is important to be aware of these limitations but also to recognize that even well-meaning health and human service professionals can possess similar liabilities. In short, an awareness of these potential liabilities may increase the likelihood of viewing CHWs as valuable community resources that must be more carefully examined and understood if their contributions to the community are to be adequately reinforced (Young, 1990).

In sum, CHWs ought to be recognized as persons with unique characteristics and functions who are capable of providing certain types of help that professionals are not able to give within our present health and medical care systems. As community-based lay workers, they provide services that are integral to the health care system, functioning as partners with a variety of health care professionals—as individuals who complement, rather than replace, other health care staff and professionals. CHWs possess unique talents, skills, and interests, offering increased potential for large time and energy investments to meet the needs of the target population (Larson, 1992).

CHWs: Program Structures and Training

Program Support Structures

CHW programs can in part be distinguished by their institutional support structures. Nearly 75% of all currently organized CHW programs throughout the nation are community-based, educational outreach services for a defined geographical community. The other 25% provide services based in and supported through state health departments, followed by schools and hospitals, and, finally, universities or colleges. This proportion is nearly replicated in the CHW programs of southern New Mexico. In addition, financial support of CHW programs is both a public and a private endeavor. Nationally, one half of all CHW programs are funded through federal or state government support, 14% are funded exclusively through private foundations and agencies, and the other third are supported through combined government (state and federal) and private funding (Brownstein & Wilson, 1994). In the rural areas of southern New Mexico/west Texas, *promotora* projects are similarly funded, with the trend toward less government support and more support from private agencies and foundations. In truth, these programs face the same competitive challenges for health care dollars and resources that other rural areas of the nation confront.

Program Structure and Goals

Successful CHW programs are well planned and are structured on clearly defined objectives. Program structural concerns include selection of CHWs; volunteer versus paid positions; strong community and health system support; adequate training and supervision; specific, understandable, and obtainable goals and objectives; and measurable evaluation criteria. Program oversight is provided by CHW coordinators. These individuals are critical for supervising, monitoring, training, and evaluating the CHW program and community health outreach workers. Without such coordinators, effective communication between the health care staff and the CHW staff is impossible.

The primary mission of most CHW programs is to emphasize prevention efforts aimed at improving health and minimizing disease, injury, and death (INMED, 1993). Current prevention efforts are determined in part by funding agencies, national and state legislative priorities, the goals of sponsoring institutions, and, at times, identified community-based needs. In the southwestern United States, CHWs focus primarily on maternal-child health-related areas, prenatal care, adolescent sexual behavior, and nutrition education. In addition, some programs address heart disease, cholesterol, high blood pressure, diabetes screening, education and follow-up, smoking prevention, child abuse, HIV/AIDS, and violence on a periodic basis. To illustrate, in southern New Mexico, several *promotora* projects (e.g., La Clinica de Familia *promotora* project in Anthony, New Mexico) are organized around maternal-child health councils that coordinate and oversee the delivery of prenatal education and care in a specified area. Membership on these councils varies but can include *promotoras,* project coordinators, public health officials and practitioners, government representatives, and health care providers. Although maternal and child health is the unifying theme, other programs that complement this theme and contribute to maternal and child health are also addressed (Barnes, 1995).

CHW Recruitment and Training

As front-line workers, CHWs are recruited from and should be trained within their communities (Woodruff, 1994). Typical recruitment strategies include referrals (54.6%), word of mouth (33.9%), community agencies (33%), and advertisements (26.5%). Across the nation, initial training for CHWs involves on average 40 or more hours. Regular in-service training is 2 to 4 hours per month, with over half (55.6%) of all CHWs receiving a certificate of completed training (Brownstein & Wilson, 1994). Recruitment and training programs in southern New Mexico/west Texas fit this national norm. In southern New Mexico, the completion of CHW training is celebrated with a graduation ceremony open to family, friends, and the community. The *promotora* project coordinator of La Familia Unida, in collaboration with others, coordinates the training of local *promotoras* and arranges this event. Such celebrations provide public recognition of accomplishment and can serve to increase the status and visibility of the *promotora* in her community.

The content and form of the education and training of CHWs must specifically address project goals. CHWs are best educated by local professionals and, when possible, in community settings. CHWs are typically trained and provided with ongoing in-service training under the direction of the CHW coordinator. These CHW coordinators are often professionally trained and may be certified health educators, licensed nurses and social workers, and/or other persons possessing specialized health-related degrees (Barnes, 1995; Brownstein & Wilson, 1994).

Curricula should reflect the most current medical knowledge in a manner that is appropriate for the learner. Educators and trainers need adequate time to prepare materials that are relevant and culturally appropriate to the community (Quillian, 1993; Swider & McElmurry, 1990; Werner & Bower, 1995; Witmer, Seifer, Finocchio, Leslie, & O'Neill, 1995). Larson (1992) recommended that the orientation training of CHWs include training about proper documentation and maintenance of client confidentiality, general knowledge (of the population, geographic area, health priorities, and community resources), cultural awareness, time management, communication, referrals, networking, safety, and documentation.

Education and training that are interactive are the most effective for CHWs (Fairbanks, 1993; Quillian, 1993; Swider & McElmurry, 1990; Werner & Bower, 1995). Problem-based learning theory can provide the basics for interactive, student-centered learning that promotes self-esteem. When education of CHWs is traditional, such as lecture-format, it should be followed with opportunities for CHW group interaction through case studies and role playing (Fairbanks, 1993).

In sum, CHWs have been shown to improve access, improve quality of care, and reduce health care costs (Witmer et al., 1995). They have potential to empower communities toward more locally controlled health planning and decision making. However, the personal challenge to the individual CHW is often great. CHWs can feel overwhelmed in this environment if they are not properly trained and prepared for the experience and can experience significant personal stress and burnout. These stresses can lead to high turnover rates. CHWs are retained best by relevant and stimulating initial and ongoing training, clear job descriptions, support from fellow CHWs and supervisors, meaningful relationships with co-workers and clients, follow-up, meeting of perceived needs, salary/incentives/benefits, and the perception of being important to the organization or clients (Brownstein & Wilson, 1994).

The Constellation of Roles

The following two major sections of the chapter examine the work of *promotoras* in the borderlands area of southern New Mexico/west Texas from a public health perspective and then from a communication perspective. Within each disciplinary paradigm, the multiple roles of *promotoras* and the consequences of those role enactments are discussed. Brief descriptions of these roles from each disciplinary perspective are provided below.

Understanding Promotoras From a Public Health Perspective

Within a public health paradigm, the *promotoras* are fundamental to prevention efforts aimed at improving the health of disadvantaged populations in southern New Mexico and west Texas. *Promotoras* link disease prevention to specific health practices through the enactment of the following roles: lay health educator, lay health care referral source, health practice role model, and social support provider. Within these roles, the *promotoras* address a variety of public health issues. *Promotoras* identify persons in need, guide them through the available health and social services system, and encourage these individuals to care better for themselves and their families. Further, as members of the community operating within the bonds of affiliation, CHWs provide informal and spontaneous assistance, advice, emotional support, and tangible aid to members of their community. Specific outreach activities of CHWs may include transporting clients, posting flyers, translating, and helping clients complete forms for services. CHWs may also conduct home visits, make educational presentations to the public and professional groups, facilitate focus groups, assist in health screening activities, represent the health service providers at meetings and conferences, and organize and carry out field assessments (Larson, 1992).

The Promotora as Lay Health Educator

Health education is a process in which relevant health information is disseminated to individuals, who can then use the information to reduce health risks and to increase the effectiveness of their health care (Kreps, 1990a). A health educator may use a wide variety of strategies for disseminating the information and may use multiple channels for communicating the information. CHWs represent an informal but directed health education effort (Kreps, 1990a). CHWs trained in appropriate health practices and disease prevention communicate this information to their clients in an informal setting, usually one on one. In this one-to-one teaching relationship based on trust and rapport, new concepts can be readily introduced while the culturally approved health beliefs and meanings of the client are maintained. Further, the client can be actively involved in the learning process with the freedom to interact within the interpersonal relationship.

Promotoras, as indigenous health educators, should value the significance of preventing illness, disability, and disease rather than relying on the more traditional model of curing disease. That is, the *promotora* emphasizes the client's healthy knowledge, skills, attitudes, and behaviors and works to develop enhanced well-being for the client. The dissemination of health information by *promotoras* may result in the empowerment of the individuals and communities that they serve. The links between information, education, and community and individual empowerment can be seen in a recent example from the *promotora* experience.

In a recent evaluation of the effectiveness of a prenatal outreach project along the Mexico/Arizona border, CHWs were shown to be highly effective in educating migrant farmworkers. Pregnant and parenting women clients reported that education in their native language in proper nutrition, exercise, and the process of labor and delivery as provided by the CHWs was very important to them. Clients also reported that the *promotoras* were their friends from whom they sought advice on subjects other than health (Warrick, Wood, Meister, & de Zapien, 1992).

Many studies have reported the changes in the *promotoras* themselves as they become the "health experts" among their peers. CHWs experience increased employment opportunities, educational advancement, increased self-esteem, and satisfaction (Warrick et al., 1992). They have contributed to the community's ability to solve its own problems. They are frequently seen as community spokespersons and have active roles beyond educator. *Promotoras* have been effective in getting funding for more police and fire protection and adequate lighting for streets. They are frequently seen as possessing valuable knowledge, and their advice is sought on these and other community activities (S. Sapien, La Familia Unida *promotora* project coordinator, personal communication, 1995).

The *Promotora* as Lay Health Care Referral Source

An important goal of some *promotora* projects in the southern New Mexico/west Texas area is to link community members to the existing health and human services system. An unfortunate characteristic of rural, poor communities is not necessarily the lack of access to health and social services but the lack of knowing which services and outlets are available within a community. Improving the knowledge of and access to such services requires establishing trust and understanding and the ability to address cultural and linguistic differences in the process of making referrals. For example, cultural beliefs about the causes and cures for particular illnesses and about who should treat those illnesses also may be personal, self-limiting factors in accessing health care resources. One such example of *promotoras* assisting in health care referrals along the U.S.-Mexico border takes into account these cultural views. For some persons of Hispanic heritage, the aid of the *curandero*[2] is essential to successful treatment of illness. Similarly, for some Native Americans, belief in the powers of a medicine man is significant for their well-being. Both of these health and social welfare providers are respected among a select group of citizens, but these same citizens are often suspicious of "Westernized" health professionals and health clinics (Geist, 1994). *Promotoras* have long experienced success in acknowledging and valuing the care of *curanderos,* medicine men, or the like while successfully promoting the services and the care that can be provided by "health professionals" of the general society. Thus, the scientific model of treatment has been successfully reconciled with the traditional, culturally based ways of healing.

In addition to these efforts to increase access to health and human service systems, *promotoras* at times function as intermediaries between individual community members and those systems. With her knowledge of the system components, the *promotora* is positioned to act as an ombudsperson for those less familiar with the procedures and structures of the system. Further, the *promotora* can advocate for community issues. Where possible, she can become a grassroots organizer, as in the developing community example described above. In other cases, she can lobby for services and training that serve her community's needs. In this respect, the *promotora* serves as the voice for those whose voice has been muted through lack of access to economic, social, and political power.

In general, efforts toward the successful integration of this underserved population into the health care system are laudatory. However, some concern has been expressed recently about the use of CHWs as client recruiters for managed-care entities. The potential for altering the nature of community health work and for diminishing the trust of community members in the CHW exists within this development. This activity should be carefully monitored and treated with caution. If this trend continues, enhanced consumer skills also ought to be advocated by *promotoras* among the communities they serve. In this way, community members will be empowered to make informed choices about their health care delivery sources.

The *Promotora* as Health Practice Role Model

As highly visible members of their communities, *promotoras* become health practice role models both for clients in the individual homes they visit and for the community at large. Their presence is felt in public gatherings and is acknowledged as having influence throughout the community. In short, the personal health habits and practices of *promotoras* are on display and are subject to evaluation by all members of the community.

Many *promotoras* have become powerful role models for smoking cessation, weight management, and injury prevention (S. Sapien, La Familia Unida *promotora* project coordinator, personal communication, 1995). Successful behavior change often requires intense follow-up, strategic plans for relapse, and strong social and/or emotional support. Fortunately, *promotoras* often can spend more time, provide more consistent and regular follow-up, and provide more intense social and emotional support than traditional health professionals can.

Another characteristic that accentuates the opportunity to be a role model for healthy behavior is the common and effective practice of home visiting. Home visiting allows the *promotora* to offer informal and spontaneous assistance in behavioral change, to provide personal advice and strategies for change that she herself has used, and to give emotional support during the process of change. Simultaneously, the *promotora* represents a powerful model of those actual changes and behaviors in her own life and is a powerful symbol of the ability to change one's behaviors and circumstances. In addition, through her wide connections in the community, the *promotora* is equipped to aid the client in making connections to others in the community who are also seeking improved health practices.

The *Promotora* as Social Support Provider

For members of a social network, social support has been defined as a system of relationships capable of providing the resources that produce mastery, provide guidance and feedback, and increase competence for the client (Caplan, 1974). As significant members of a client's network, *promotoras* help their clients to achieve these ends through the provision of support. As *promotoras* enter the homes and lives of their clients, they form relationships with the women, men, and children they serve. Within these relationships, they provide support of three primary types: instrumental, informational, and emotional (House & Cottington, 1986).

Instrumental support is defined as the exchange of time, resources, and/or labor (House & Cottington, 1986). This kind of support is often seen as tangible assistance toward the accomplishment of goals (Albrecht & Adelman, 1987). In southern New Mexico/west Texas, many *promotora* projects focus on maternal and child health. Aiding new mothers, especially teen mothers, in acquiring parenting skills is a priority. In this effort, the *promotora* frequently spends time in the home helping to care for the infant, simultaneously teaching infant care techniques, modeling those behaviors, and offering some short-term relief to the new mother. *Promotoras* have also been known to assist with Lamaze techniques during labor and delivery for the young mother when the boyfriend or parents refuse assistance.

For example, in Doña Ana County, New Mexico, the Welcome Baby Program of New Generation of Family Services, Inc. provides support at no charge to new mothers through the work of trained volunteers. Visits to first-time mothers begin before the birth of the baby and continue for 12 months following birth. Through home visits and phone calls, the *promotora* volunteer provides aid and education to the new mother, emphasizing the importance of parent-child bonding and age-appropriate stimulation for the infant (L. Bracey, personal communication, 1996).

The second type of support, *informational support,* has been defined as the general provision of information about a variety of issues (House & Cottington, 1986). For example, the *promotora* may provide important information about disease prevention, immunizations, or the health care system and resources available, as described for the lay health educator role. Just as important, the *promotora* may provide informal training in communication skills or problem-solving skills. This skill training serves the community member in all aspects of his or her life. For example, a *promotora* may offer information about strategies for dealing with a rebellious teen or an abusive husband.

Finally, *emotional support* is described as empathy, caring, love, and trust (House & Cottington, 1986). Statements of reassurance and acceptance are communicated to recipients by the support provider. When *promotoras* engage in relationships with their clients, they create a bond of trust. This trust is enhanced by the fact that the support is coming from a person who is similar to the client (i.e., homophilous relationship; Rogers, 1983; Rogers & Kincaid, 1981). When the *promotora* enters a home, she may find multiple problems. Often issues of domestic violence, marital conflict, or disciplinary problems with children are brought to the attention of the *promotora* by the client. Although these problems may require that *all* of the *promotora's* skills be brought to bear, a central skill in this effort is the provision of emotional support for clients who are severely distressed. In sum, the *promotora* becomes a peer counselor for the client. In an environment with few services, where neighbors may live far apart and where daily life is a struggle, this support is critical.

In sum, in their public health role enactments, CHWs become catalysts for change by promoting grassroots community efforts and enabling individual empowerment. CHWs aid communities and individuals in developing and adopting strategies appropriate to coping with the problems they face (Moore, 1990). In the day-to-day practice of these public health roles, CHWs aid individual community members and the community as a whole to gain confidence and some measure of control over their own lives.

Understanding Promotoras *From a Communication Perspective*

Within a communication paradigm, the *promotoras* can be described as participants in formal and informal networks of communication. Within these networks, significant communicative functions and roles can be identified. In network terms, *promotoras* are simultaneously group members and intergroup linkers. In other words, they have significant amounts of communication with other members within a group and also serve to bind two or more groups together, thus moving messages from group to group. As a consequence of this simultaneous membership and group identification, *promotoras* enact the following network roles: opinion leader, gatekeeper, bridge, and liaison. The performance of these roles suggests that *promotoras* exhibit the following communicative strengths: (a) an ability to persuade and influence members of their own network and members of other networks; (b) the communicative complexity to control information flow among members of the network and the skill to modify messages in a variety of ways and to filter messages from one member to another; (c) the capacity to connect a network to the broader environment via the reciprocal processes of information gathering and dissemination; and, finally, (d) a willingness to create and negotiate linkages between and among diverse networks.

In sum, through their communication network role performances, the *promotoras* become empowered and become a source of empowerment for developing healthy individuals, families, neighborhoods, and communities.

The *Promotora* as Opinion Leader

As defined by network analysts, an opinion leader is an informal leader within the social system in which he or she exerts influence. Such an individual does not hold a formal position and hence does not wield power and influence associated with that formal authority, but nonetheless has the ability to guide and influence the other members of the network (Kreps, 1990b). In a sense, these individuals are "magnetic centers" who draw people to them for information and advice (Walton, 1963). The leadership of these individuals is acquired and maintained through demonstration of their technical competence and their social accessibility (Rogers, 1983). Further, opinion leaders demonstrate a conformity to the system's existing norms and may lose their degree of influence over and respect from other system members if they deviate too far from the system norms. To be effective, opinion leaders must be viewed by other community members as "of the system," not apart from it. By their close conformity to the system's norms, opinion leaders serve as an excellent model for the innovation behavior of their followers (Katz & Lazarsfeld, 1955; Rogers, 1983).

The most significant characteristic of opinion leaders is their influential position within their system's communication structure: They are at the center of interpersonal communication networks. The importance of this role as opinion leader and communication center can be illustrated by an example from a recent meeting of CHWs from across the state of New Mexico. The focus of the meeting was a discussion of strategies for retaining CHWs and increasing their career opportunities. Preliminary to the discussion, the CHWs were discussing some of the stresses they faced in their work. Several of these women mentioned that they were "on call, day and night" for the members of their communities. Some described clients who sought them out at home for advice, support, and assistance. Though the stress of these demands on CHWs is clear, equally clear is the significance and value of these women to the persons whose lives they touch.

The *Promotora* as Gatekeeper

A gatekeeper in a communication network controls the flow of information through the network. Located in the middle of the communication network, the gatekeeper is the recipient of large amounts of information. He or she prioritizes the information, determines the appropriate recipients for some or all of the information, and conveys that information to the recipients (Kreps, 1990b). In this process, the gatekeeper also can serve translation and filtration functions. That is, the gatekeeper will first of all sort through the information and decide what is relevant to which members of the community served. Then the gatekeeper engages in a translation of the information such that congruence with the language patterns, meaning structures, and beliefs about speaking (topics for discussion, who should speak, where, when, etc.) of the clients is assured (Hymes, 1974; Philipsen, 1989). For the *promotora,* initial and ongoing training programs provide a solid information base that is valuable to the community members being served. This public health-related information then needs to be communicated through multilingual, multifaceted modes of communication (home visits, radio, written materials). Indeed, the *promotora* often must exhibit a very high level of personal competence in communication in that she must have at her disposal a wide range of communication strategies from which to select and then enact, depending on the needs of a particular client (Fisher, 1986).

This formal information acquisition and consequent reframing within the community experience can be demonstrated in diabetes screening and education. The rates of diabetes among the populations served by the *promotoras* is higher than national averages. Some *promotora* projects are aimed specifically at this disease; others include diabetes within the many health problems of the community served. Regardless, *promotoras* are often given training in this disease and its management.

Whereas medical management of some of these cases is required, in other cases changes in lifestyle and diet can help to manage this chronic disease. However, diet and lifestyle are rooted in the cultural, social, and economic conditions of the individual. Thus, the trained *promotora* as a participant in those context conditions can translate her medically based information into the frameworks of meaning held by the members of her community who have this disease or who may be at risk for diabetes.

The *Promotora* as Bridge

A bridge is an individual in the network who is a member of one clique (i.e., a group of individuals who communicate more frequently with one another than with other network members) who connects the clique to the members of other cliques. Within this bridge role, the individual functions as a conduit or channel for the exchange of information. First, the bridge is able to pass information from his or her membership group to other groups. Conversely, the bridge serves to gather information from other groups and bring it into his or her clique. In the case of *promotoras,* the health worker is a community member who knows and understands the community. She connects the community, both formally and informally, to outside groups. For example, some *promotora* projects in southern New Mexico/west Texas are affiliated with nonprofit health care agencies. These agencies provide formal instruction and training in health-related information to the *promotora,* which she then "channels" into her community. Within these agencies, the *promotora* also has informal information exchanges with her sister CHWs serving other communities and informal exchanges with the coordinators of the program, health care providers, and other agency representatives. These informal interactions can provide insights and strategies that are transferable and useful in her own community. In reverse, the *promotora* is able to present the perspective of her community to these various groups. Some *promotoras* are deeply involved in needs assessment strategies within their communities. These grassroots-level evaluations of community strengths and weaknesses provide a pool of information for other groups, such as public health agencies and legislative bodies, to use in developing program priorities. Further, these CHWs are repositories of knowledge and information about community beliefs, attitudes, and mores. This information would be much more difficult for traditional health care providers to access. Such "insider" information is vital to successful program development and implementation in that the *promotora* can offer insights about the utility and meaningfulness of particular interventions planned for her community.

The *Promotora* as Liaison

The concept of liaison refers to a role in the network that functions to link two or more groups or cliques (Farace, Monge, & Russell, 1977; Kreps, 1990b). As a member of neither of the linked groups, the liaison provides the objectivity of an outsider while connecting two entities whose efforts require coordination and a certain degree of cooperation. In this role, liaisons are perceived as having influence. That is, because they have a level of power, they can exert influence to bring two groups together. Further, in the process of linking the groups, that perception of influence is increased.

Because of their many contacts within and beyond the community, *promotoras* can function as a primary point of contact when various groups wish to connect with other groups in the borderlands. An example from recent efforts by university personnel to conduct a study of exposure to hantavirus and to provide prevention information and education about this disease to underserved populations (see Chapter 4 of this book) serves to illustrate.

Persons who live in rural areas or who are engaged in agricultural work are particularly vulnerable to this illness. Further, these individuals are less likely to have access to the necessary information about simple precautions that can be taken to limit exposure to the virus. Thus, the outreach efforts represented in the *promotora* project seemed an ideal venue to initiate this work. Contact was made with a *promotora* group in Luna County of southern New Mexico. After the researchers had developed a relationship with the *promotora,* her cooperation and support was gained for the project. The university researchers expressed a desire to do similar hantavirus exposure evaluations and prevention and education in the sister community, Palomas, across the border in Mexico. The *promotora* then linked the university researchers with the mayor of this village and other village government officials. This mayor was helpful and supportive of the project. In short, the liaison role of the *promotora* linked university and local government entities and provided a cooperative link to other communities.

Promotoras also serve this linking function in indirect ways. That is, because of the increasing interest in these community health models, representatives from numerous agencies, institutions, and local, state, and federal government groups converge wherever *promotoras* meet. In these cases, the CHW coordinator is more likely to play the liaison role when the management of the contacts between these various groups and the *promotora* groups themselves must be accomplished. Also, the linkages among these groups are often coordinated through the CHW supervisor for the purpose of a multiple-pronged approach to addressing the issues and problems identified by the *promotoras.* For example, at the CHW meeting described previously, in addition to the *promotoras* themselves, representatives from two different universities, representatives from several regional public health departments, and several national foundation grantees were among those present. All of these entities have an interest in supporting the CHW model, and the interest expressed by these agencies demonstrates a belief in the importance of these programs. Nonetheless, each entity also brings to these meetings its own agendas and viewpoints regarding the best approaches to community health problems, training, evaluation procedures, and so on. These differences and tensions are then "liaised" through CHW coordinators, who connect the groups to each other and to specific *promotora* projects.

In sum, the *promotoras* are vital communication resources, channels, and links within their communities. Further, their communication abilities are the life force of their capacity to create and sustain relationships with a wide variety of individuals and groups in the day-to-day performance of their tasks. As the "magnetic centers" of their communication networks and the performers of multiple communication role functions, these women become sources of strength and forces for change within their communities.

Promotoras as Boundary Spanners

As suggested in the introductory section of this chapter, we believe that the unifying principle of all the role enactments of the *promotoras* is boundary spanning. In network terms, a boundary spanner is an individual who is able to connect his or her interpersonal network to the "environment" (Kreps, 1990b). Clearly, CHWs enact this role in the performance of their activities as they go "beyond the borders" of their communities. Indeed, in many respects, the *promotora* is a representative example of what has become known as the "strength of weak ties" hypothesis (Granovetter, 1973). Weak-tie linkages between people are ties that may be relatively infrequent or of low intensity. These ties function to connect individuals with access to significantly different information sources. Weak ties in communication networks are important because they have the capacity to bring information to persons and groups who would not be likely to receive it (Monge & Eisenberg, 1987). This boundary spanning is clearly accomplished by CHWs. However, CHWs cross boundaries, both literally and figuratively, in other significant ways.

First, CHWs cross boundaries of age, gender, education, and social class in their role performance. They are available to aid all members of their communities. They work with the young and the elderly, with men and with women, with those in desperate poverty and with those living on the edge of poverty. CHWs also coordinate their efforts with individuals whose economic status and educational attainment are higher than their own. This boundary spanning is valued for the insights that these workers provide on ways to best raise the health status of underserved, often hard-to-reach populations. In fact, *promotora* networks work best when CHWs from a particular community respond to community-focused health-related and health care needs while coordinating services with health and human service professionals.

In another view of boundary spanning, the boundaries and constraints of definitions of health and illness in a community are reexamined by community members with the aid of *promotoras*. While preserving the integrity of culturally based health, illness, and treatment beliefs, CHWs introduce new health-related information into their communities and new strategies for approaching these health problems. In addition, CHWs help their communities to redefine some of their economic and social conditions in terms of factors that influence the health, well-being, and overall development of their communities.

Finally, the disciplinary and research boundaries of public health and communication paradigms are crossed within an examination of *promotoras* programs. Though calls for crossing the boundaries of disciplinary paradigms abound, such boundary spanning is not the vogue. Renewed efforts to identify common interests and diverse approaches not only can lead to greater energy in addressing social problems but also can broaden our understandings of those problems. *Promotoras* projects present a valuable opportunity for crossing boundaries within the academy that then allows us to cross the boundaries between the academy and the community in collaboration with the community.

Notes

1. It is interesting to note that the *promotoras* of southern New Mexico are all women. However, CHWs in other areas of the country and the world may be either male or female. For example, CHWs in Mexico and in South America can be male or female and are called *promotores,* a non-gender-specific term. Though one might argue that characteristics of the cultural milieu along the U.S.-Mexico border determine the gender singularity of CHWs in this region, we simply do not have enough data or compelling evidence to draw such a conclusion. Indeed, an equally viable explanation for women only as *promotoras* can be found within the needs assessed and the funding supporting these programs initially. In southern New

Mexico, identified community needs included maternal and child health, teen pregnancy, and domestic violence. Funding sources supported these women's health issues. Further, these women's health-related issues suggested to early organizers of the programs that women in the role of *promotoras* would be more effective with the population at issue.

2. *Curanderismo* is a folk-healing belief system widely adhered to among Hispanic populations. The belief system supports the treatment of a variety of illnesses with a combination of mild herbs, psychosocial interventions, and religion. The *curandero* is the practitioner of these folk-healing arts. For a further discussion of this issue, see, for example, Chesney, Thompson, Guevara, Vela, and Schorrstaedt (1980), Comas-Diaz (1989), and Geist (1994).

References

Albrecht, T. L., & Adelman, M. B. (1987). *Communicating social support.* Newbury Park, CA: Sage.

Barnes, M. D. (1995). *The development of recommendations for a community health worker* (promotora) *education and training program.* Las Cruces: New Mexico Department of Health, Public Health Division, New Mexico Border Health Office.

Brownstein, J. N., & Wilson, K. M. (1994, November). *Community health advisors.* Paper presented at the American Public Health Association Community Health Advisor Special Public Interest Group, Washington, DC.

Caplan, G. (1974). *Support systems and community mental health.* New York: Behavioral Publications.

Centers for Disease Control and Prevention. (1994a). *Community health advisors: Vol. 1. Models, research, and practice: Selected annotations—United States.* Atlanta: U.S. Department of Health and Human Services, Public Health Service, Centers for Disease Control and Prevention.

Centers for Disease Control and Prevention. (1994b). *Community health advisors: Vol. 2. Programs in the United States: Health promotion and disease prevention.* Atlanta: U.S. Department of Health and Human Services, Public Health Service, Centers for Disease Control and Prevention.

Chesney, A. P., Thompson, B. L., Guevara, A., Vela, A., & Schorrstaedt, M. F. (1980). Mexican-American folk medicine: Implications for the family physician. *Journal for Family Practice, 11,* 567-574.

Comas-Diaz, L. (1989). Culturally relevant issues and treatment implications for Hispanics. In D. R. Kowlow & E. P. Salett (Eds.), *Crossing cultures in mental health* (pp. 31-48). Washington, DC: Sietar.

Fairbanks, J. (1993). *Case studies in reaching out: A training manual for community health workers in New Mexico.* Albuquerque: University of New Mexico, Prenatal Care Network.

Farace, R. V., Monge, P. R., & Russell, H. M. (1977). *Communicating and organizing.* Reading, MA: Addison-Wesley.

Fisher, B. A. (1986). Leadership: When does the difference make the difference? In R. Hirokawa & M. S. Poole (Eds.), *Communication and group decision making* (pp. 197-215). Beverly Hills, CA: Sage.

Geist, P. (1994). Negotiating cultural understanding in health care communication. In L. A. Samovar & R. E. Porter (Eds.), *Intercultural communication: A reader* (pp. 311-321). Belmont, CA: Wadsworth.

Gottleib, B. H. (1985). Social networks and social support: An overview of research, practice, and policy implications. *Health Education Quarterly, 12*(1), 5-22.

Granovetter, M. (1973). The strength of weak ties. *American Journal of Sociology, 78,* 1360-1380.

House, R. J., & Cottington, E. (1986). Health and the workplace. In D. Aiken & D. Mechanic (Eds.), *Application of social science to clinical medicine and health policy.* New Brunswick, NJ: Rutgers University Press.

Hymes, D. (1974). *Foundations in sociolinguistics: An ethnographic approach.* Philadelphia: University of Pennsylvania Press.

International Medical Services for Health. (1993). *Opening doors for healthier families: A guide for resource mothers. Resource mothers' handbook.* Sterling, VA: Author.

Katz, E., & Lazarsfeld, P. (1955). *Personal influence: The part played by the people in the flow of mass communication.* New York: Free Press.

Kreps, G. L. (1990a). Communication and health education. In E. B. Ray & L. Donohew (Eds.), *Communication and health* (pp. 187-203). Hillsdale, NJ: Lawrence Erlbaum.

Kreps, G. L. (1990b). *Organizational communication* (2nd ed.). New York: Longman.

Larson, K. (1992). Excerpts from community outreach guidance: Strategy for reaching migrant and seasonal farmworkers. *Migrant Health Clinical Supplement, 9*(5), 3.

Monge, P., & Eisenberg, E. (1987). Emerging communication networks. In F. M. Jablin, L. L. Putnam, K. H. Roberts, & L. W. Porter (Eds.), *Handbook of organizational communication: An interdisciplinary perspective* (pp. 304-342). Newbury Park, CA: Sage.

Moore, G. F. (1990). A catalyst who inspires self-help: The community health worker in deprived areas. *Community Development, 5,* 342-344.

Office of Migrant Health. (1992). *Community outreach guidance: A strategy for reaching migrant and seasonal farmworkers.* Washington, DC: U.S. Department of Health and Human Services.

Ortega, H. H. (1992). *Present trends and future possibilities of health along the United States-Mexico border.* El Paso, TX: Pan American Health Organization.

Philipsen, G. (1989). An ethnographic approach to communication studies. In B. Dervin, L. Grossberg, B. J. O'Keefe, & E. Wartella (Eds.), *Rethinking communication: Paradigm exemplars* (pp. 258-269). Newbury Park, CA: Sage.

Quillian, J. P. (1993). Community health workers and primary health care in Honduras. *Journal of the American Academy of Nurse Practitioners, 5,* 219-225.

Rogers, E. M. (1983). *Diffusion of innovations* (4th ed.). New York: Free Press.

Rogers, E. M., & Kincaid, D. L. (1981). *Communication networks: Toward a new paradigm for research.* New York: Free Press.

Steckler, A. B., Dawson, L., Israel, B. A., & Eng, E. (1993). Community health development: An overview of works of Guy W. Steuart. *Health Education Quarterly, 20,* (Suppl. 1), 3-27.

Swider, S. M., & McElmurry, B. J. (1990). A women's health perspective in primary health care: A nursing and community health worker demonstration project in urban America. *Family Community Health, 13*(3), 1-17.

U.S. General Accounting Office. (1990). *Home visiting: A promise for early intervention strategy for at-risk families* (GAO HRD-90-83). Washington, DC: Author.

Walker, M. H. (1994). *Building bridges: Community health outreach worker programs.* New York: United Hospital Fund of New York.

Walton, F. (1963). *A magnetic theory of communication* (NOTS Pub. No. 3). China Lake, CA: Naval Ordinance Test Station.

Warrick, L. H., Wood, A. H., Meister, J. S., & de Zapien, J. G. (1992). Evaluation of a peer health worker prenatal outreach and education program for Hispanic farmworker families. *Journal of Community Health, 17*(1), 13-20.

Werner, D., & Bower, B. (1995). *Helping health workers learn.* Palo Alto, CA: Hesperian Foundation.

Witmer, A., Seifer, S., Finocchio, L., Leslie, J., & O'Neill, E. (1995). Community health workers: Integral members of the health care work force. *American Journal of Public Health, 85,* 1055-1058.

Woodruff, S. (1994). Community health advisors to begin training in pilot project. *Arizona Area Health Education Centers Newsletter, 8*(1), 8.

Young, R. (1990). Lay health advisors: Who they are and why they are an important health intervention strategy. *Migrant lay health advisors: A strategy for health promotion* (Vol. 1). Chapel Hill, NC: Department of Maternal and Child Health.

Chapter 10

⁣∽∾⁣

PROJECT VIDA

Community Health Models That Work

BILL SCHLESINGER

Project Vida is a multiple-social service agency sponsored by the Presbyterian Church USA (PCUSA) and the Cumberland Presbyterian Church. It has been developed as part of a strategy to respond to the unique and overwhelming needs and possibilities in an area of cultural encounter and exchange. Though church sponsored, Project Vida is community based. Its programs and priorities have been developed through the concerns and issues presented by the community around it. It does not require formal religious activities as a condition or aim of its services.

El Paso is approximately 70% Hispanic and is the fifth poorest metropolitan area (Standard Metropolitan Statistical Area) in Texas. The population of the focus area is about 12,000, and that of the service area is 45,000. Project Vida's service area is located immediately on the U.S.-Mexico border and is a primary port of entry for legal and undocumented persons. Ninety-nine percent of those living in the service area are of Hispanic ethnicity. The median yearly income in the focus area is less than $7,000 for a family of four, rising to about $14,000 in the wider service area. The median age in the focus area is 15 years. In 1993, the area had three times the violent crime rate of the city (7 crimes per 1,000 persons vs. 2 per 1,000 persons a year). Gangs are a part of the community social system, and many have continuous existence over three or four generations. Sixty-five percent of the adults (25 and older) have less than a ninth-grade education. Housing is dilapidated and overcrowded; over 500 families in the service area are "doubled up" in apartments or single-family homes. Employment in the traditional garment industry has been shrinking as a result of operations' moving to Mexico and other parts of the world.

The entire service area is a federally designated medically underserved area (MUA) and a health professional shortage area (HPSA). About 70% of the families have no medical insurance. The county hospital, R. E. Thomason General Hospital, is located within the service area and is about six blocks from the focus area. Clinics at the adjacent Texas Tech Health Science Center have a 3-month waiting list for appointments. As a result, the emergency department has been historically used for primary care for families and children. Families have at best pieced together disjointed services. They have had to travel 7 miles on a very limited public transportation system to receive Women, Infant, and Children (WIC) services.

Project Vida conducted interviews in 100 homes in the winter and spring of 1989 to develop an initial community assessment. Beginning in the fall of 1989, Project Vida worked with La Mujer Obrera, an advocacy and service organization for garment industry workers, to establish a volunteer-driven clinic in their center. In the fall of 1990, Project Vida moved into a small duplex near the center of the focus area and obtained funding for a physician's assistant to provide full-time family clinic services under physician supervision. Community residents became involved first as visitors, then as volunteers. Five community residents conducted extensive interviews with over 100 households in 1991. Faculty at the University of Texas at El Paso (UTEP) School of Nursing and Allied Health helped develop a questionnaire and tabulated results. Also in 1991, the first annual Community Congress was held, where low-income families who were registered with Project Vida met to review and evaluate programs and build priorities for future development. These congresses are held in a local elementary school cafeteria. Normally about 100 adults attend and participate in each congress.

Broad-based programs emerging from the interviews and the congress meetings include health, housing, gang prevention, and education. Health programs include health education in homes and at central locations provided by *promotoras* (community health promoters), a food-buying co-op, a bilingual licensed family therapist, developmental pediatric consultations, an optical program for buying prescription eyeglasses, home visitation of newborns for enrollment in Early Prevention, Screening, Diagnosis, and Treatment (EPSDT) and monitoring of immunization, the development of a family practice clinic served primarily by midlevel practitioners, and an outreach home visitation program for families using the emergency room for pediatric primary care. Housing programs have addressed the lack of affordable, safe housing in the area by the construction of 20 apartment units, with more on the way. Families living in unsafe conditions can receive services from a homelessness prevention program with social workers who help them with monitoring and reporting environmental hazards and who provide renters with training and advocacy for their rights and responsibilities as tenants. Gang prevention has included development of an after-school program for 50 children a day that includes field trips, tutoring, crafts, dance, and cooperative games. Education has included preschool classes, a one-on-one reading program for early elementary school children that offers them the incentive of buying Christmas presents for their families and teachers if they complete certain levels of participation, a multimedia computer lab, and adult education classes (English as a second language, GED, and citizenship).

Innovation

Project Vida's programs focus on involving families in increasing control of and responsibility for their own future. Little is "given." A thrift shop charges nominal prices for clothing and household goods. Children earn credits that allow them to buy presents for their families. Parents buy new jackets and Christmas gifts for $3 rather than having them donated directly to the children. The eight apartments built by Project Vida and the 12 now under contract for construction have a small fenced yard for each unit, allowing a sense of control and ownership of space.

Project Vida's programs are interconnected. It is normal for a family to come to the clinic, attend a health education presentation, shop in the thrift shop or food co-op, and have a child in a preschool class and a parent in the English as a second language class. Such interconnectedness facilitates working with a whole family and gives staff a way to evaluate needs and problems with help from a variety of disciplines. Families are "known" and become part of the network of care as they, in turn, help others.

Project Vida began by working with the community to help it define its own vision, then went on to develop programs that made that vision real, and finally involved other agencies as "partners" in the process. In so doing, it found ways to solve joint problems cooperatively.

El Paso City/County Health District (EPCCHD) was providing prenatal care in the area but had no facilities to provide primary care for the mother or her family. Project Vida's space was very limited in its small building. The health district agreed to lease its clinic building in the community to Project Vida at no cost for evening primary care and agreed to refer primary care to Project Vida and accept referrals for prenatal care. This was the first such agreement to share space by the health district, which has since led to the health district's contracting with other providers. Project Vida now provides space for the WIC program to serve clients, eliminating a 7-mile trip for many of them.

As part of the city/county's Immunization Action Plan (IAP), Project Vida proposed receiving the birth records of newborn infants in its service area from the county hospital. An outreach worker and case manager coordinate visits to the families of the newborn infants, offering registration and follow-up for immunization and EPSDT services. Families who accept services are offered a full variety of support services directly or by referral, based on their case management plan.

Thomason Hospital's emergency department (ED) records indicated that the ED was often used to provide primary care for children. An average of 500 families used it two or three times a year for nonemergency pediatric purposes. This was poor primary care as well as costly for the hospital system. The planning department of Thomason Hospital and Project Vida proposed funding for a nurse case manager and a community outreach worker to visit families using the ED for pediatric care. The program was put in place in January 1995. A release form is offered to families in the ED. Those who sign (almost 100%) are referred by fax on a weekly basis to Project Vida. The nurse case manager and the outreach worker attempt to contact the families through home visits (about 50% of the addresses are valid; others are nonexistent or families have never lived there or have moved). An initial assessment by the visitor with the family discusses why the ED was used and offers alternatives and support. If the family is willing, the nurse case manager develops a case management plan with them and follows up.

Case management plans have included getting heat in an apartment during the winter and teaching mothers how to read thermometers and use fever suppressants appropriately. They have included enrollment in Project Vida's primary care clinic, family counseling, transportation services, and a variety of other needs that directly affect the health of the child and the family.

Collaboration

In addition to the city/county health district and Thomason Hospital's ED, Project Vida has negotiated low-cost laboratory services with Thomason Hospital's lab. It is a participant in joint El Paso Title V funding for medical services for women and children not covered under any other program. It is contracted with WIC to provide space for weekly services. It is a "charter member" of the El Paso Cancer Consortium, which provides early detection services to uninsured women and men, to fund Project Vida's clinical breast and prostate exams and referrals for mammography. Project Vida is a member of the Sun Country Recreation Collaborative, which coordinates the city's summer recreation program and provides support for Project Vida's program for 50 children, which is offered at the local elementary school. It is a member of the El Paso Coalition for the Homeless and has received their support in obtaining funds to begin a transitional living center and build additional permanent housing. It also provides services to residents of the Salvation Army's Transitional Living Center and Emergency Shelter. Project Vida is a member of the Family Pride Coalition, which has been funded by the Texas Children's Defense Fund to provide parenting and preventive education for children; the project provides parenting education services as part of that program. Zavala Elementary School regularly makes space available for Project Vida's programs at no charge and refers children to Project Vida for services. The UTEP School of Nursing and Allied Health sends advanced nurse practitioner students to Project Vida for clinical training, with our staff serving as preceptors or training faculty for the students. Project Vida also serves as a research site for the UTEP School of Public Health. It provides work sites for older citizens under Project Ayuda. It is an AmeriCorps site and is finishing its fifth and final year as a VISTA project. Project Vida coordinates programs with La Mujer Obrera, the El Paso Interreligious Sponsoring Organization (EPISO, a community organizing project), the Coalition for Affordable Housing, and others.

Outcomes

About 1,300 families are registered with Project Vida, and the primary health care clinic sees about 350 patients a month who would otherwise have no primary care service. Ninety-seven percent of the infants and children registered with Project Vida's programs are on schedule for immunizations, compared to 70% citywide. Out of 81 births during the last year under case management, 4 newborns weighed under 5 pounds and none under 3.7 pounds. This means none of the infants were considered "high risk."

Only 3 of the 250 families contacted by the program have returned to the ED at Thomason, and all three of those cases have been appropriate use (broken arm, very high fever during the night, and severe scalp laceration). In addition, clients report a greater sense of control of their own family, less of a sense of helplessness, and satisfaction with being able to use basic health care tools and procedures.

If 250 families had used the ED three times during the year for primary care, cost to the county hospital would have been $262,500 at $350 per visit. Cost for the primary health care clinic is $48 per visit. The same 250 families visiting the clinic cost $36,000. The cost for the outreach program is $70,000. For a total cost of $106,000, the program saves over twice that much in expenses.

Individual and group evaluation conversations have reported several factors that seem related to sociopsychological changes: (a) The use of noninstitutional buildings was perceived by some individuals as making a more "homelike" atmosphere; (b) clients who became volunteers almost uniformly reported decreased anxiety concerning their own circumstances and an increased sense of ability to deal with their own needs as a result of becoming involved with the needs of others; and (c) clients who reported a perceived change in their ability to cope with their situations reported a sense of direct human concern from Project Vida staff separate from any specific "help" and reported a general welcoming and respect as part of the overall atmosphere in Project Vida.

Project Governance and Structure

PCUSA and the Cumberland Presbyterian Church both use a strongly representational system of governance. Assemblies of lay and clergy representatives make decisions at all levels of each denomination, and a great deal of their work is done in lay/clergy committees. The board of Project Vida is named by committees of both denominations on the basis of local board recommendations (one member from the Cumberland Presbyterian

Church, the balance from PCUSA). These include persons who are clients and recommended from the local community. The midlevel governing body of PCUSA is the Presbytery of Tres Rios. This is the most attentive governing body and provides much of the core funding for administration, as well as access to local churches for additional support. It is responsible for naming the PCUSA board members. The board of Project Vida functionally reports to the Mission Committee of the Presbytery of Tres Rios. In addition to the corporate structure of Project Vida, there is a "daughter" corporation, PV Community Development Corporation, that handles housing and facilities development activities. It is a recognized community housing development organization (CHDO) and receives federal funding from the Department of Housing and Urban Development for its projects through the City of El Paso. Though many board members overlap, it has one-third community representation.

Internally, Project Vida functions with a strong codirector team who are also husband and wife and ordained Presbyterian clergy. Each program area—health, housing, education, gang prevention—has a staff leadership team that works in coordination with the codirectors. Volunteers, Ameri-Corps members, and staff are integrated in program teams. An administrative group—bookkeeper, clerk, service tracking and billing person, and secretary—works under the direction of the codirectors and with each program area. A weekly staff meeting unites all the program areas in a general review and planning session that deals with agencywide issues and concerns. General staff training includes group planning and reflection methods.

Replication and Sustainability

Project Vida has proposed the ED outreach model to two of the for-profit hospitals based on an initial charge per referral, additional charges for registering and serving the referred patient in its clinic, and a rebate if the patient returns to the hospital for nonemergency care. The proposals are currently under review.

Project Vida is not unique in any of its individual services but is striking in its integration both horizontally and vertically (Figure 10.1). It follows the model of "locality development"—an approach highly suited to the "one-stop shopping" health care approach. This approach is sustainable in a variety of resource settings. It depends on coordination among private and public partners with the community's vision of its own future and skilled facilitation of that process. Portions of the programs may expand or disappear depending on local support, availability of funds, and availability of skills and resources. But the approach allows use of a variety of resources and community support. To date, funds have not been a limiting factor in the program's sustainability.

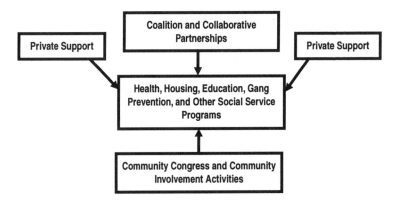

Figure 10.1. Model of Project Vida's Locality Development Approach

This model can be adapted for any community where practitioners are free to invest time in community visits and to adapt or develop programs without traditional boundaries on the types of services or staffing patterns required. It is most suited to smaller agencies, but its participatory methods can be used in larger organizations where top management is committed to its support.

Chapter 11

✌︎∽✍︎

ALTERNATIVE APPROACHES TO HEROIN TREATMENT AND AIDS PREVENTION AMONG YOUTH IN A MEXICAN BORDER CITY

REBECA L. RAMOS
JOÃO B. FERREIRA-PINTO
MARIA E. RAMOS

The main objective of this chapter is to describe the stepwise growth process of two drug rehabilitation and treatment interventions designed to help decrease the rate of heroin usage while preventing the spread of AIDS among injecting drug users (IDUs) in Ciudad Juárez, Mexico. The organic development of the program, Compañeros, from a research demonstration program to a full-fledged community-based organization (CBO) will be described, as well as the changes in the treatment approach reflecting changes in available resources. The first intervention discussed, which we refer to as Intervention A, targeted the general intravenous-drug-using (IDU) population in Juárez, and the second, which we will refer to as Intervention B, concentrated its recruitment efforts among adolescents and young adult users of heroin and cocaine between the ages of 13 and 21. Specific approaches dealing with problems facing drug-using adolescents

AUTHORS' NOTE: This research was funded by grants from the Mexican Health Foundation (FUNSALUD), Mexico, D.F., and the Levi Strauss Foundation, San Francisco, in cooperation with the U.S.-Mexico Border Health Association (USMBHA), El Paso, TX.

and their families will also be discussed. To make it easier to describe and compare, this chapter will concentrate on participants in both interventions between 13 and 21 years of age.

The theoretical perspective of the development of the intervention strategies will also be discussed, and examples of the content matter presented to the youth population will be described. Preliminary findings of a comparison of the results of both strategies in the areas of client participation and the self-reported change in drug usage will also be discussed. The main contribution of this chapter is the documentation of the development of a CBO drug treatment program in a changing environment and the discussion of the decision-making process involved in maintaining a quality program with very scarce resources. It is our contention that the interventions described here can very easily be adapted to similar populations living in other communities on the U.S.-Mexico border and in other regions in the United States other than the border—especially those communities that suffer the same lack of resources as the border region.

Background

The 6 million people who live in counties that are contiguous to the U.S.-Mexico border have very similar socioeconomic, cultural, and health profiles. On both sides of the border, they are young, poor, subject to a number of infectious diseases, and, in high numbers, medically indigent (Ferreira-Pinto, Ramos, & Shedlin, 1996). The majority are of Mexican descent. These border populations also share a high degree of illegal drug usage aggravated by the lack of affordable drug treatment services. This is especially true in the urbanized regions that comprise the Tijuana-San Diego and the Ciudad Juárez-El Paso trade corridors.

Among these two main corridors, the cities of Ciudad Juárez-El Paso make up the largest urban complex on the border, and are the oldest, the most active, and perhaps the primary point for heroin shipment into the United States. In the past, these distribution channels ended in the main drug wholesale markets of Houston, Los Angeles, Chicago, and New York, but recently, with the increase in the detection and apprehension rate in larger cities, smaller cities "such as St. Louis, whose heroin supply previously came from Los Angeles, now receive shipments [directly] from . . . Texas border towns" (National Institute on Drug Abuse [NIDA], 1994, p. 27). This high level of trade in heroin has as a primary consequence the artificially high rate of monetary growth in the local economy of El Paso and Juárez, with a parallel increase in crime and official corruption. It also has a very serious secondary consequence: The increase in the rate of drug availability and the decrease in drug prices increase the opportunities for young people to experiment with drugs. The abundance of heroin in the border area, coupled with a lack of resources for law enforcement, has in a few decades transformed Juárez into the city with the highest level of heroin consumption in all Mexico (Tapia-Conyer, 1994).

In the 1994 *Encuesta Sobre el Consumo de Drogas en la Frontera Norte de Mexico* ("Survey of Drug Consumption on the Border of Northern Mexico"; Tapia-Conyer, 1994), the Direccion General de Epidemiologia (Director General of Epidemiology) sampled cities on the northern border of Mexico to establish a baseline for studying the changes in incidence and prevalence rates of drug use among the general population in four cities: Tijuana, Ciudad Juárez, Monterrey, and Matamoros. The prevalence rate among those who answered affirmatively to the question "Have you ever used any illegal drugs?" was 10.1% in Tijuana, 8.9% in Ciudad Juárez, 5.8% in Matamoros, and 2.8% in Monterrey. Interestingly, heroin use was not reported in Matamoros or Monterrey, and its reported use was higher in Juárez (0.8%) than in Tijuana (0.6%). The same pattern of higher prevalence in Juárez (1.1%) than in Tijuana (0.6%) was also reported for inhalants (Tapia-Conyer, 1994).

The high level of heroin usage in Juárez is not easily detectable because users tend to engage in their drug-using behavior in secluded locations or in their homes or the homes of friends. But indirect measures, such as the numbers of users seeking treatment, the numbers of deaths from overdose, the number of arrests for drug possession, and other indicators, can be used to estimate the level of consumption. Employing the number of users seeking treatment as one of the indicators uncovered a "hidden" population of heroin users during the latest attempt by the U.S. Immigration and Naturalization Service (INS) to stem the northern migration of Mexican workers looking for jobs in the United States. When a blockade along 12 miles of the Juárez-El Paso border was established, it successfully decreased the number of people crossing illegally into the urban area of El Paso but had an unexpected secondary effect: It created a shortage of heroin available to drug users in Juárez.

Before the blockade, many Mexican heroin users had crossed the border daily to buy the drug because they believed that the quality was better and that they had more reliable U.S. sources for obtaining the drug (Ferreira-Pinto et al., 1996). The heroin shortage caused by the blockade, coupled with the recent devaluation of Mexican currency, made it much more expensive to acquire heroin in Juárez. This increase in the monetary and transaction cost of obtaining the drug led to an increase in the number of users who sought treatment because they could not afford the same level of drug use any longer. What would have been a success in a more affluent community—heroin users voluntarily coming to treatment centers—became a problem to the already underfunded Juárez treatment facilities (Ramos & Ferreira-Pinto, 1996). The problem of diminishing treatment resources and increased demand does not affect Juárez alone. In El Paso, as in many U.S. cities, there has been a decrease in the number of treatment centers and a corresponding increase in the number of users who have been waiting to obtain a treatment slot in a rehabilitation program.

The decrease in the level of funding for drug treatment programs also affects the search for more efficacious drug treatment modalities. Diminishing resources do not allow for programs to provide researchers and government officials with the necessary data for evaluating program outcomes, the comparison of the results of the few treatment modalities available, or research on the composition and special needs of drug-using subpopulations. It also impedes the creation of longitudinal databases necessary to evaluate the possible impact of drug treatment efforts in a community.

Besides the lack of reliable data needed for research, little progress has been made in the study of the differences and similarities among drug-using subpopulations. There is a lack of published applied research on drugs in the border region that can be used by program managers trying to develop treatment and prevention programs that take into consideration the peculiar binational character of the region. Furthermore, the small amount of data that has been collected and reported officially is not altogether reliable. For instance, the number of IDUs reported by the Epidemiology of Addictions Surveillance System (SISVEA) in Juárez is much smaller than the summation of the data compiled by outreach workers and treatment facilities and reported to the local health department in Juárez (Ferreira-Pinto et al., 1996). The same is true when one tries to collect information about the prevalence of heroin use in El Paso from the Texas Commission on Alcohol and Drug Abuse (TCADA). Since 1995, lack of funding to treatment programs other than methadone clinics has removed the leverage that TCADA had in requesting El Paso treatment providers to report the number of drug users under their care.

Besides the lack of reliable epidemiological data on drug use, there is a lack of information about the particular patterns of initiation, progression, and cessation of drug use among Mexican populations. The few research projects on drug use among populations of Mexican descent have used theoretical constructs about drug initiation, progression, and cessation based on findings generated from other drug-using populations in the United States, without taking into consideration the variety of subcultures present in the population. Many studies have recommended that interventions for change should be concentrated in the areas of interpersonal relationships, family, school, and social circles (Hawkins, Jenson, & Catalano, 1987; Leavit, 1995) but have failed to take into consideration the special circumstances of the U.S.-Mexico border environment and the lack of trained people that would be needed to accomplish the proposed intervention designs.

These studies concentrated on acculturated Mexican Americans who had largely adopted the mores of the dominant Euro-American culture. The most commonly cited "Tecato" (heroin user of Mexican descent) study focuses on a Mexican American heroin subculture whose epicenter is Los Angeles. In this study, Mata and Jorquez (1988) stated that Tecatos rely heavily on social networks to guide them in the initiation of drug use and progression toward addiction. The authors also reiterated the common assumption—that most Tecatos share a belief system—*la vida loca,* or "the crazy life." This and other studies (Moore, 1994; Moore & Vigil, 1987; Vigil, 1988) have been confined to the United States and conducted in cities far away from the U.S.-Mexico border. Many of the prevention strategies recommended by the Center for Substance Abuse Prevention (CSAP), for instance, have been designed on the basis of research conducted among acculturated Latinos. Specific treatment strategies that may be applicable to recent arrivals into the United States have not been described (CSAP, 1994).

The interventions described in this chapter attempt to address this research gap by adapting a number of accepted treatment modalities while taking into account the cultural idiosyncrasies of this particular population of heroin users. These interventions are the distillation of the experiences and the applied knowledge of a number of researchers who during the last decade have been attempting to find culturally relevant and cost-effective ways to deal with the problems of drug abuse and AIDS on the northern Mexican border. Although the prevalence of AIDS cases among drug users in Juárez is low according to official statistics, the same problem of lack of reliable epidemiological data about drug usage is also present in the AIDS statistics. Only scattered anecdotal evidence is currently available. For instance, during the first months of 1996, five cases of possible pediatric AIDS were brought to Compañeros for treatment, of which three were from HIV-positive mothers whose partners were heroin users. The treatment programs described in this chapter could be easily adapted to other communities in the border region or to communities in other U.S. regions with a large population of Mexican migrant workers.

Historical Overview of the Compañeros Drug Rehabilitation Strategies

A brief chronological description of the evolution of the interventions can shed some light on the background of the intervention strategies and on how a CBO (Compañeros A.C.) has used its limited resources to create a cost-effective treatment program for heroin users in Juárez. Given its origin as an HIV prevention research program, Compañeros has made HIV prevention one of the mainstays of the treatment program. Since 1989, the program has established an AIDS clinic, which, to this day, is the only treatment facility available to indigent HIV patients in Juárez.

June 1987 to December 1990

The drug rehabilitation program started in 1987 as a small pilot for a NIDA multisite research grant on prevention of HIV transmission among female sexual partners of heroin users. NIDA decided to fund this project in Mexico for comparison with other Latino populations in the United States and because of the border region permeability to drugs and drug users. One cannot think of the border as a real barrier; it is a political demarcation to which the inhabitants of the region pay little heed. The interests of NIDA in the region were scientific and also pragmatic: There is the possibility of disease being transmitted between drug-using populations on both sides of the border.

The initial needs assessment among IDU partners showed the need for the development of a center where detoxification and rehabilitation could be provided for heroin users and their families. As part of the final stages of the research, such a center was established in Juárez. From 1987 to 1990, heroin detoxification was accomplished using painkillers under medical supervision. At this stage, there was minimal use of support groups for the heroin user or his or her family, apart from the meetings between the IDUs and the medical doctors and nurses and occasionally a psychology intern from the local university. It was a minimal operation, with the financing for the drugs and medical personnel donated by the Pan American Health Organization field office and maintained by the overhead generated from other studies being conducted by Compañeros staff.

January 1991 to September 1993

In January 1991, a grant from the Levi Strauss Foundation allowed the program to start a full-fledged drug treatment program based on a model developed and used with success by the Lincoln Hospital in New York City. This treatment is based on the use of sterilized needles placed in specific acupuncture points in the patient's ears to help decrease pain and create a sense of well-being. The acupuncture treatment was supplemented by a number of Chinese herbal medicinal preparations to which were added less expensive traditional Mexican medicinal teas. It took time and lots of convincing for the Mexican heroin user to accept and trust the acupuncture treatment. We speculate that the use of needles was, symbolically, the cause for the initial discomfort, given that the participants had long experience with needles. The medical staff working on the new acupuncture protocol were helped in their efforts to detoxify their patients by the synergetic work being done with the female sexual partners of the IDUs, who were enrolled in a concurrent demonstration research project financed by NIDA.

Counseling for the individual heroin users and their families was very limited in the first year of the new program, but during this time, the staff of Compañeros managed to establish a Narcotics Anonymous (NA) group in Ciudad Juárez. Although there has been fluctuation in the number of participants in this NA group, mainly due to drug use relapse, the group has not disbanded and continues to this day as the only NA group in the city. The final evaluation of this project demonstrated that the lack of an electronically based management information system (MIS) makes it difficult to do a rigorous evaluation of the efficacy of the treatment, which anecdotal evidence demonstrated to be very successful. An extension of the first grant was obtained from the Levi Strauss Foundation with the explicit task of developing a research-based MIS for Compañeros.

October 1993 to December 1994

During this period, a new data collection system was developed, field tested, and implemented. The system allowed for better documentation and analysis of program process and outcomes. It also allowed the program staff to identify easily and rapidly intervention strategies that appeared to improve rehabilitation, evaluate these strategies, document and improve on those strategies that were useful, and discontinue or modify unsuccessful strategies. The facility to assess the progress of the interventions pointed to some modifications that appeared necessary to improve the efficacy of the program. Among the many modifications and additions, the following were the most important:

- Encourage a more active participation of the clients and their families in the maintenance of the program's physical installations to increase the sense of ownership in the program.

- Require that clients begin to take over the provision of everyday supplies (sugar, cups, napkins, spoons, etc.) to increase their sense of responsibility for the maintenance of their program.

- Require that clients "pay back" part of their treatment by "working" 4 hours a week for the program. Two of these hours could be used to attend the NA sessions.

- Instruct the clients and their families to conceptualize and accept the basis of the treatment program: (a) the treatment has three components: acupuncture, counseling, and support group; (b) attendance at all three components is imperative for treatment success; and (c) the treatment does not stop at the end of 6 months but is a continuous process of vigilance engaged in by clients and their families against situations that might bring about a relapse.

January 1995 to June 1996

One of the main findings in the analysis of outcome data between 1993 and 1994 was that although there was a decrease in the number of users seeking treatment who were younger than 15 years, there was an increase in the number of clients who stated that they had started using heroin before they were 15 years old. The program was reaching users only after they had spent a number of years injecting drugs and had been exposed to a number of highly infectious diseases, including tuberculosis, hepatitis B, and HIV. With the support of the Mexican Health Foundation (FUNSA-LUD) and the Carnegie Corporation, an intervention targeted to adolescents and the young adult male IDU population (Intervention B) was designed and implemented.

Detailed Description of the Interventions

Both interventions, A and B, are based on a combination of health promotion and treatment models, such as the health belief model (Hochbaum, 1958; Rosenstock, 1974), social cognitive theory (Bandura, 1986), the harm reduction model (O'Hare, Newcombe, Matthews, Buning, & Drucker, 1992), and the stages-of-change model (Prochaska & DiClemente, 1983; Prochaska, DiClemente, & Norcross, 1992). These models are described elsewhere and we will only briefly discuss the stages-of-change model. These models have been slightly modified and adapted to a heroin-using population and to the socioeconomic and cultural realities of a Mexican border population.

When the participant is first admitted to the program, a rapid assessment, using the stages-of-change approach, is made to gauge his or her readiness to engage in the heroin rehabilitation program. The stages-of-change model (Prochaska et al., 1992) posits that individuals are in different stages of the change process at different times in their addictive careers. The initial stage is one of precontemplation, in which there is no desire for change; the second stage is one of contemplation, in which the thought of change crosses the mind of the addict; the third stage is one of preparation, during which the individual makes a decision to change; the next stage is the action stage, in which the individual acts on his or her decision and joins a detoxification program, for example; and the last stage is one of maintenance, in which the addict works to stays off the drug. Patients arrive at the program mostly in the preparation or action stage, although in some cases the participant has been "persuaded" by family and friends to come into the program and may not be prepared to start treatment. This initial assessment of the participant "stage" in the rehabilitation process is used as a guideline for the choice of the strategy that will work best for each participant. During the first 2 weeks of the program, the main principles of the health belief model and the social cognitive theories are used extensively. Information is continuously provided to increase the participants' perception of their susceptibility and the consequences of the possible contagion with a number of serious infirmities that can be brought about by episodes of drug injection. The participant is not only warned of the dangers but made to realize that he or she can avoid these dangers and that the necessary tools and the skills to use them will be made available during the course of the treatment. During these first weeks, there are discussions about the barriers that have prevented the participant from attempting to stop using drugs in the past, and skills are taught to help overcome them. These barriers are quite different for adults and for adolescents, and the program staff emphasizes the most salient barriers to overcome for each intervention group.

In Intervention B, the young participant is presented with information about the risks and susceptibility to diseases from an adolescent's perspective. Problems such as peer pressure and other barriers to recovery and relapse prevention that are typical of adolescents are emphasized. Adolescents in possession of this information and the skills necessary to avoid relapse will, it is hoped, engage in less risky behaviors and at a much lower rate than adolescents who did not have this training. It is also hoped that they will have a lower rate of relapse after recovery.

Compañeros' harm reduction philosophy was developed after many years of observation of the cyclical pattern of detoxification, cessation of use, relapse, drug usage, and search for treatment. It is the staff's experience that this cyclical pattern will eventually stop, but meanwhile the best approach is to keep the user from acquiring some lethal disease. The program's harm reduction approach stresses that although abstinence is the most effective way to avoid problems associated with drug use, success in treatment cannot be measured only in terms of complete and total abstinence, with no episodes of relapse. The harm reduction approach strives for a change toward the safest possible behavior while using drugs and an incremental weaning away from the drug until complete abstinence is achieved. Success is measured by the degree to which an individual is at less risk for encountering the problems occasioned by drug use and by how well the user becomes integrated or reintegrated into the community after the detoxification and at the end of the rehabilitation process. The focus is on the long-term gradual change of behavior toward full recovery, which implies abstinence.

In both A and B interventions, the individual treatment is divided into four components: (a) physical (the acupuncture treatment), (b) psychological (counseling), (c) family (family support groups), and (d) social (support groups for the participant). The first two components of the intervention have remained constant since 1991 and are present in both interventions. The main difference is the orientation of the family and social components: During Intervention A, the discussions take an older adult perspective on problems (parenting, financial problems, jobs, etc.), whereas during Intervention B, the discussion themes have a youth point of view and deal with adolescent concerns (dating, peer pressure, school, etc.).

Physical Component

Since their inception, the treatment services provided by Compañeros have contained detoxification and maintenance regimes that include acupuncture and herbal medication. The selection of these strategies was made in consultation with NIDA's Community Research Branch and was based on clinical trial findings that showed that the protocol of the Lincoln Hospital in the Bronx, New York, was cost-effective and successful in the treatment of heroin addiction. The Compañeros program staff obtained free training from Lincoln Hospital staff in the detoxification and maintenance regimes, including the use of auricular acupuncture and the use of traditional Chinese herbal medicine. The high cost of Chinese herbs, coupled with high Mexican importing duties, forced the program to search for less expensive substitutes for its medicinal herbs. After studying the literature, searching in medical electronic databases, searching the Internet, and interviewing medical herbs experts on both sides of the border, one of us managed to find equivalent herbs (such as valerian and chamomile)[1] whose medicinal effects are similar to those of the costly Chinese herbs used in the teas served to program patients.

The typical rehabilitation process takes from 1 to 6 months. On the day of admission, and daily for 2 whole weeks, the patient is given between 45 to 60 minutes of acupuncture treatment (the longer session is used after the patient gets used to the acupuncture needles) followed by the ingestion of two or three cups of an herbal tea combination. The patient is also given tea bags and vitamin pills to take at home, with instructions on how to prepare the tea and when to take it together with the vitamins. An intravenous solution containing vitamins, iron, and calcium is given to the patient whenever the attending physician recommends it, but especially on Fridays. This intravenous application appears to help the patients maintain a drug-free status during the 2-day weekend while the program is closed.

After the first 2 weeks, the patient is moved into a maintenance regime, which consists of the same steps delineated above but administered only once a week. This regime may continue for 6 or more months until the patient and counselor decide that only an occasional "booster" session is needed. Patients are also strongly encouraged and are given incentives to attend the support groups and NA sessions to help them cope with their new drug-free lifestyle and to help avoid recidivism. One of the main points that is continuously stressed during the program is the avoidance of the risky behaviors and situations that can lead to exposure to HIV infection, especially sharing needles and patronizing former drug-based hangouts and social networks.

Psychological Component

During the admission process, the participant is given general information about the program detoxification and maintenance components and also a thorough explanation of the biological, psychological, and social aspects of addiction. This is a long process that may last from 1 to 2 hours, depending on the formal educational level of the participant. Following this, on the same day, the patient is given a general physical exam and, if necessary, is directed to other organizations in Juárez that have reciprocal referral arrangements with Compañeros for housing, specialized medical care, spiritual support, and more intensive psychological counseling.

On the second or third day of the program, a needs assessment is done, and, on the basis of the initial medical and psychological diagnosis, a treatment plan is prescribed and a counselor assigned to the client. An analysis is conducted of the obstacles and protective factors affecting the particular participant. Strategies to combat barriers and reinforce protective factors are also discussed with the client. In subsequent sessions, the participant is given an explanation about HIV infection and counseling on HIV prevention, including the dangers of needle sharing and unsafe sex. Participants are strongly encouraged to have an HIV test done for their own protection and the protection of their sexual partners. If the participant is interested, he or she is given an HIV pretesting counseling session explaining all the procedures involved in the testing and results reporting.

Lack of funds has motivated the redesign of the psychological component. During Intervention A, the psychological component is delivered by a clinical psychologist, but for Intervention B, the counseling is limited to crisis intervention and to HIV pre- and posttest counseling. The counselors are social workers who have received short-term training in crisis intervention and extensive training in HIV pre- and posttest counseling and the treatment theories used in the program.

Family Component

The program strategy calls for the treatment to concentrate on the participant as part of a family unit and stresses the role of family members in the rehabilitation process. Although 80% of the participants are 21 years of age or older, their families—especially their mothers, even more than their sexual partners—influence the outcome of the treatment. To use these very powerful allies, the program requires the participation of the family in support groups and in counseling sessions. Although fewer than 10% of the participants are brought into treatment by a family member, after a while the participants recognize the importance of their family as part of the treatment and become allies of the program by recruiting their families to become joint participants in the rehabilitation process.

We have found that when a participant's family is encouraged to participate in the program, two patterns appear: (a) They wholeheartedly join the program efforts and start acting as "spies" for the program and keeping the participant "in line," or (b) they reject the invitation and take the attitude that the program should "fix" the participant and return him or her to the family "cured." When this happens, family members are quickly made to understand that the treatment is a "family affair" and that their participation in the support groups is vital and required for the success of the program and the participant's rehabilitation. The family component is a crucial part of the process, and a special curriculum has been created for the family support group. The curriculum deals with the following themes, among others, and what should be done about each of them:

- Heroin addiction and withdrawal syndrome
- Other family members' attitudes toward addiction
- Emotional support favorable to rehabilitation
- Overdosing
- Relapse signals
- Mental health and mental disease symptoms
- Prevention of drug dependence among other family members
- Relationship between drugs and HIV and prevention of HIV

Although we have not formally measured changes in family members' attitudes, after regular attendance at the support groups we can detect a change in their attitudes toward drugs. For instance, the word *vice* is no longer being used and is replaced by *illness,* the pressure on the client to quit immediately decreases, and there is a preoccupation with preventing other members of the family from becoming involved with drugs. This appears to happen regardless of the degree of progress of the client.

The family members most commonly in attendance during Intervention A are the wife or sexual partner of the participant. For Intervention B, the most common family representative is the mother or a mother surrogate (grandmother, aunt, or adoptive parent). One of us refers to the occasional father that accompanies the participant as a surrogate mother because in most of these instances a mother is not present in the household, and the father takes that role during treatment and in many other areas of the participant's life.

Social Component

Given the lack of resources, the program cannot concentrate its efforts on a community-level intervention. But within the counseling and group sessions, a microcosm of the social environment of the addict is created, examined, and critically analyzed by the counselor. The teaching of critical thinking guidelines to these participants is still in an initial phase, but the changes that have occurred are encouraging. For instance, one of the participants stole a small tape recorder used to play soothing music during the acupuncture sessions. After analyzing what he had done and recognizing the damage he had caused to the program's participants and staff, he returned the tape player and apologized for the theft. He has become one of the most helpful volunteers in the program and has been abstinent for about 2 years.

The group sessions for Intervention A are open to all program participants, and the barriers to recovery are discussed without taking into consideration the age of the client. According to the theme list in the curriculum for group sessions, the topics discussed for Intervention A are adult centered (see Appendix B). For example, when the topic of the family is discussed, the emphasis is on existing marital relationships. The group sessions for Intervention B focus on adolescent participation, and special care is taken to encourage participants between the ages of 13 and 20 to attend. During these sessions, topics that are of relevance to adolescents and young adults are discussed (see Appendix C). Topics of daily life such as school, relationships, partner selection, and the relationship between parents and children are emphasized. This approach also helps older participants to improve their relationship with their own children and to decrease one of the causes of stress in their own lives.

For Intervention B, two basic modifications have been made to the design of the sessions: (a) The felt or perceived needs of adolescents in the behavioral, cognitive, emotional, and social aspects of their lives are recognized, and (b) during the sessions, success on the road to recovery is

TABLE 11.1 Age of the Target Population in Interventions A and B

Age	Group A		Group B	
	No. of Cases	*% of Cases*	*No. of Cases*	*% of Cases*
< 14	5	7.7	5	9.4
15-17	18	27.7	29	54.7
18-20	42	64.6	19	35.8

measured using the harm reduction approach—the less drug one consumes, the closer one is to the complete abstinence from the drug.

Because the majority of the young users in Group B have been using multiple drugs, the emphasis of the program is to reduce the number and then the quantity of drugs being consumed, to refrain from taking risks for contracting HIV (i.e., using injectable drugs), and to change gradually their network of friends by replacing friends who use drugs with friends who do not. These social component sessions take place after the acupuncture session and last between 1 and 3 hours. Attendance at the group session is voluntary, but participants are strongly encouraged to attend.

Preliminary Results of the Interventions

Although the final comparative evaluations of the results of the interventions are not yet available, a number of indicators point to some success in the adolescent target group enrolled in Intervention B. The adolescents attending the two groups were not completely comparable in age, although they were similar in a number of other characteristics. For example, Table 11.1 shows that although the majority of participants in both interventions were between the ages of 15 and 20 years old, the youngest cohort (individuals younger than 14) was represented by only 7.7% of the population in Intervention A and by 9.4% in Intervention B. The trend in Intervention B is toward younger participants.

Over 80% of either group had never married, and approximately 13% were currently either married or in common-law relationships (see Table 11.2). Only 20% of Intervention A participants were employed in a permanent full-time job, whereas 24% of Intervention B participants were employed. In Intervention A, 72.3% were underemployed, in contrast to 64%

TABLE 11.2 Marital Status

	Group A		Group B	
Marital Status	No. of Cases	% of Cases	No. of Cases	% of Cases
Single	54	83.08	45	86.54
Married	6	9.23	2	3.85
Common-law	3	4.62	5	9.62
Sep./divorced	2	3.08	2	3.85

TABLE 11.3 Drug Use Decrease Before and After Intervention

	Group A			Group B		
Drug	No. of Initial Users	No. Using Less	% of Decrease	No. of Initial Users	No. Using Less	% of Decrease
Marijuana	51	37	72.5	29	24	82.8
Sedatives	39	35	89.7	24	14	58.3
Heroin	37	28	75.7	22	15	68.2
Cocaine	34	28	82.4	19	17	89.5
Inhalants	15	13	86.7	14	10	71.4
Speedball	8	6	75.0	7	6	85.7
Stimulants	4	4	100.0	1	1	100.0
Hallucinogens	0	0	0.0	0	0	0.0
Crack	1	0	0.0	1	1	100.0

in Intervention B. The percentage of students was 7.7% in Intervention A and 13% in Intervention B participants.

Drug Use Patterns Before and After

All the enrollees in both interventions used multiple drugs (Table 11.3). In a follow-up interview at 6 months after enrollment, a pattern of decrease

TABLE 11.4 Number of Participants Attending Counseling and Group Sessions

No. of Sessions	Group A				Group B			
	Ind.	%	Group	%	Ind.	%	Group	%
None	12	18.5	21	32.3	34	61.8	25	45.5
1-54	26	4.6	33	50.8	15	27.3	22	40.0
6-10	11	16.9	6	9.2	6	10.9	2	3.6
11-15	0	0.0	2	3.1	0	0.0	5	9.1
16-20	0	0.0	2	3.1	0	0.0	1	1.8
>21	0	0.0	1	1.5	0	0.0	0	0.0

in drug use was observed for both interventions. The drug consumption is presented as a percentage in the decrease of use for each type of drug. There is a decrease in the number of users for all drugs except crack cocaine in Intervention A, but given that we detected only one crack user among Intervention A participants, this is not a significant result.

Changes in rate of consumption are self-reported and are not based on a blood exam or urinalysis. Both tests are expensive and beyond the financial capabilities of a CBO in Juárez. Given that Compañeros does not use a "punitive" approach for dealing with drug users and that the staff have a high level of sensitivity, we believe that these self-reports obtained during face-to-face interviews are reliable.

Participation in the Interventions

Participation in intervention activities was similar for both interventions (see Table 11.4), and there is a progressive decrease in the number of sessions attended over the course of the treatment. Both individual and group sessions show a larger number of participants attending one to five sessions and then dropping out. This pattern is not atypical in most therapies, in which the average number of sessions attended is four. The number of participants in sessions was, overall, greater among participants in Intervention A, with 51% of the participants attending one to five sessions compared to 40% of the participants in Intervention B. However, between 12% and 13% of participants in Groups A and B, respectively, participated in between 6 and 15 sessions.

Although the participation in the individual and group sessions appears to be less among the participants in Intervention B, the overall number of adolescents and young adults seeking and participating in rehabilitation services increased from 2.8 per month to an average of 6.5 per month. With the introduction of youth-oriented activities, there was an overall increase of over 200% in the number of youth served. This has to be tempered by the overall increase in clients of all ages during the time that Intervention B was going on; this increase was only on the order of 27%, with the number of new clients enrolled in the program jumping from 15 to 19 participants per month.

Conclusion

Given that we have not conducted the final comparative evaluation of the interventions, the conclusions we can draw from the above are very general. It seems that both interventions made a difference in the lives of the participants and that the new adolescent-based intervention has been successful in attracting the type of adolescent IDUs who have not commonly placed themselves in risky situations and who can be helped to understand that abstinence from drugs is necessary for their own well-being and that of their families. The decrease in the use of drugs appears to be the trend among adolescents who participated in Intervention B, which offers strategies that are easy to use to prevent relapse. However, the most eloquent testimonies to the potential benefits of interventions come from individuals that have participated in them. These are the testimonies of two participants.

El Muerto (The Dead One), 45 Years Old, Participated in Intervention A:

> I started using drugs because I had $1 on me. Some friends needed an extra dollar to be able to afford their doses. They injected me with some drops, and I started using it. But then I decided to stop for a while when I started vomiting, feeling lousy, and falling all over the place. I could not eat. When I stopped, I started feeling even worse [*la malilla,* withdrawal], and I asked some friends what was the problem, and I was told that if I injected again, the pain would pass. I did it and I felt "cured," and I liked it.
>
> I have been coming to Compañeros for 1 year and 2 months. The program has really worked for me. It took about 10 days for me to fully feel the effects of the program, but there are also a lot of feelings associated

with the drug that I have to fight constantly. I wish I could erase from my mind the feeling of dependence on a few drops. Without the Compañeros program, I believe I would still be shooting heroin. I was brought in by a friend, and I have also brought in many of my friends. One thing that helps a lot is that the program is free. When one is under the influence of the drug, one can get the money for treatment, but when one is in treatment one has to change, and it is very hard to get any kind of money. I have been hungry because of my treatment. But I also have received a lot of support from the counselors and my support group. I feel that I have a family here in Compañeros.

Raymundo, 20 Years Old, Participated in Intervention B:

I am a heroin user. I had been using heroin for 3 years until my wife had a HIV test in Compañeros and she tested positive. My younger son had just been born. I felt terrible. First I was so disgusted with myself that I became crazy. It was the worst time of my life. I felt like a corralled bull, closed in, desperate—worse than a withdrawal.

That was when [the counselor] looked me up and convinced me to take the exam. Of course, I was also positive. That was when I decided to stop. I had double withdrawal symptoms: first the drug, and then the moral aspect—I had infected my wife and probably my two kids. I do not want them to be tested. My older son was always sickly and has some developmental problems; my younger son is very healthy. If I knew one of them was positive, I would kill myself.

I am free of drugs, thanks to the acupuncture needles and the counselors in Compañeros. My wife and I also receive HIV/AIDS treatment in the afternoon. I have become closer to God, and I ask that he help me in this hour of need.

Note

1. Valerian is one of the species of the Valerianaceae family of plants, which are central nervous system depressors. It is used as a sedative and antispasmodic. Chamomile (*Aster trifolium*) is used as a sedative.

References

Bandura, A. (1986). *Social foundations of thought and action*. Englewood Cliffs, NJ: Prentice Hall.

Center for Substance Abuse Prevention. (1994). *A Hispanic/Latino family approach to substance abuse prevention.* Rockville, MD: Author.

Ferreira-Pinto, J. B., Ramos, R. L., & Shedlin, M. (1996). Migrants and female sex workers: HIV/AIDS on the U.S. Mexico border. In S. I. Mishra, R. F. Conner, & J. R. Magaña (Eds.), *AIDS crossing borders: The spread of HIV among migrant Latinos* (pp. 113-136). Boulder, CO: Westview.

Hawkins, J. L., Jenson, D. J., & Catalano, R. (1987). Delinquents and drugs: What evidence suggests about prevention and treatment programming. In B. Brown & A. Mills (Eds.), *Youth at high risk for substance abuse.* Rockville, MD: National Institute on Drug Abuse.

Hochbaum, G. M. (1958). *Public participation in medical screening programs: A socio-psychological study* (PHS Pub. No. 572). Washington, DC: U.S. Public Health Service.

Leavit, F. (1995). *Drugs and behavior.* Thousand Oaks, CA: Sage.

Mata, A. G., & Jorquez, J. S. (1988). Mexican-American intravenous drug users' needle sharing practices: Implications for AIDS prevention. In R. J. Battjes & R. W. Pickens (Eds.), *Needle sharing among intravenous drug abusers: National and international perspectives* (NIDA Research Monograph No. 80). Rockville, MD: National Institute on Drug Abuse.

Moore, J. W. (1994). *Going down to the barrio: Homeboys and homegirls in change.* Philadelphia: Temple University Press.

Moore, J. W., & Vigil, D. (1987). Chicano gangs: Group norms and individual factors related to adult criminality. *Aztlan, 18,* 27-44.

National Institute on Drug Abuse. (1994). *Texas Epidemiologic Work Group report.* Washington, DC: Author.

O'Hare, P., Newcombe, R., Matthews, A., Buning, E. C., & Drucker, E. (Eds.). (1992). *The reduction of drug-related harm.* New York: Routledge.

Prochaska, J. O., & DiClemente, C. C. (1983). Stages and processes of self-change of smoking: Towards an integrative model of change. *Journal of Consulting and Clinical Psychology, 51,* 390-395.

Prochaska, J. O., DiClemente, C. C., & Norcross, J. C. (1992). In search of how people change: Applications to addictive behaviors. *American Psychologist, 47,* 1102-1114.

Ramos, R. L., & Ferreira-Pinto, J. B. (1996, June). *Alternativas de rehabilitacion para usuarios adolescentes de drogas inyectadas.* Paper presented at the Reunion Nacional de Investigadores, Fundacion Mexicana para la Salud (FUNSALUD) and Carnegie Corporation, Taxco, Mexico.

Rosenstock, I. M. (1974). Historical origins of the health belief model. *Health Education Monographs, 2,* 328-335.

Tapia-Conyer, R. (1994). *Encuesta sobre el consumo de drogas en la frontera norte de Mexico.* Mexico, D.F.: Direccion General de Epidemiologia, Secretaria de Salud.

Vigil, D. (1988). *Barrio gangs.* Austin: University of Texas Press.

Part 4

❧

Community and Health Promotion in the Border Region

Since the late 1980s, community has been a central theme in popular and academic discourse, giving rise to such terms as *imagined communities* and *virtual communities.* This emphasis on community was partly a response to the homogenizing influences of mass media on a global and domestic level. In the United States, however, it was also a reaction to changes in the political system of health funding and the need to focus on grassroots empowerment. Cities and states could no longer be sure of government support even though they were held accountable to deliver government requirements and standards. The focus on community in public health has a much longer history in that the significance of community participation has long been recognized as imperative to the health of its members.

In the U.S.-Mexico border region, the focus on community as a central concept is of particular importance. First, on both sides of the border, but particularly on the Mexican side, the inhabitants of the *colonias,* or substandard subdivisions, are migrants or immigrants from different regions in Mexico. They do not share an identity in terms of family networks or regional traditions. Many of their close family members still live in their home towns throughout Mexico. Second, because of the scarcity of resources, both individual and collective, it is necessary to share the limited resources that are available. To establish norms and expectations that are likely to benefit the collective, health researchers and practitioners in border regions have reinforced the value of community in the populations in which they work.

The four articles in this section emphasize the importance of community as a central organizing principle in health promotion efforts in the U.S.-Mexico border region. The authors identify the multiple obstacles encountered in achieving successful health promotion efforts built on the concept of community. Many of the challenges involved in the community-based programs require a level of trust and a belief in the value of the collective benefit. These requirements are particularly difficult to meet in populations that feel legally and economically vulnerable. There is also the constant challenge of the mobility of migrant populations that experience very little, if any, stability.

Chapter 12

⤲

NOTES ON COMMUNITY HEALTH ON THE BORDER FROM THEORY AND PRACTICE

THERESA BYRD

Working on health issues with communities is one of the most rewarding and challenging roles of public health practice. In schools of public health, nursing, social work, and allied health sciences, students are taught the importance of working "with" rather than "on" communities and are encouraged to work for the "empowerment" of communities, groups, and individuals. In this chapter, I will briefly review some of the models and theories of working in community and then, using my experience with a community-based border health project, discuss some of the challenges of working in community, especially on the U.S.-Mexico border.

Models of Community Work

It is common for health professionals to see the health problems of individuals as related to individual lifestyles, especially because chronic diseases such as cancer and heart disease have become the leading causes of death in much of the world. Clearly, there is some truth in this—we know

AUTHOR'S NOTE: Parts of this chapter, such as the description of Project Verdad, appeared in the journal *Hygie* (now *Education and Promotion*), Vol. XI, No. 4, December 1992, and are reprinted with permission.

that smoking causes cancer and that poor diet and lack of exercise lead to obesity, heart disease, and diabetes. Still, most are aware that the environment in which persons live has some impact on their health and the decisions they make about their lifestyle. Social norms, advertising and media, and accessibility and availability of health care services and information affect not only people's choices but their perception of possible choices. In many cases, people may not have choices about their health risk exposures because of unequal distribution of resources, issues of environmental equity, and lack of access to care (see Chapter 7 of this book). Although health professionals must have concern for the individual to a certain extent, it is imperative that they also be involved in community-, organization-, and policy-level change. Although all levels of change are important, this chapter will focus on the community level.

Today in the United States, there is a federal mandate for community-based programming. In the field of public health, one of the early advocates of working with communities to help them meet their health goals was Dorothy Nyswander (1967), who encouraged public health educators to "start where the people are" and to work for an "open society" where everyone would have the opportunity to reach his or her full potential. Nyswander's ideals continue in the work of many of her students. One such student, Meridith Minkler (1978, 1992), continues to research and work with communities. She and other health educators draw on the work of Paulo Freire (1970), who advocated "education for critical consciousness"—a process that encourages people to look for the problem behind the problem to develop creative and empowering solutions (see also Chapter 7 of this book). Saul Alinsky (1972) was interested in creating

> mass organizations to seize power and give it to the people; to realize the democratic dream of equality, justice, peace, co-operation, equal and full opportunities for education, full and useful employment, health, and the creation of those circumstances in which man [sic] can have the chance to live by values that give meaning to life. (p. 3)

His work has encouraged health workers to organize communities to social action.

In 1970, Jack Rothman described three models of community organization. The first he called *locality development,* in which the community is empowered to solve problems on its own. This approach is not task oriented but process oriented, in the hope that what is learned by the community will be useful in varied situations. In locality development, the health worker is seen as a facilitator—someone who helps the community discover its needs and develop solutions. Rothman's second model is the *social planning* approach, in which "experts" enter a community, diagnose the problem, and then propose a solution. The community may be, but is not necessarily involved in the diagnosis or the planning of any interventions. This is a task-oriented method that does not leave the community with skills to solve future problems and is a model often used by health agencies. In some situations, such as a disease outbreak, this is the most useful model. Unfortunately, it is commonly used in all situations, usually because it is seen as less costly and less time intensive. Many important health programs have failed because the community was never asked for its input into the planning process. Rothman's last model of community organization is called *social action*. With this approach, the outsider acts as an advocate to clarify social issues and lead the community in an effort to change their society. This describes the work of Saul Alinsky (1972) and others who were involved in the civil rights movement, the United Farmworkers movement, and, most recently, campaigns to improve the lives of people with AIDS and to develop stricter tobacco ordinances.

These models are almost never used in isolation from each other. Most community organizers blend them as they attempt to best serve both the community and the agency for which they work.

Over the years, there have been many advocates for working with communities to help them solve health and social problems. They have several common concepts about how to "empower" communities and develop health interventions that will work. These include involving the community in all aspects of planning, intervention, and evaluation; working with communities on the needs that they feel are most important; and organizing communities in such a way that they can learn the process of working together to solve common problems. The question for many practitioners is exactly *how* this can be accomplished.

The next section of this chapter will describe one project based in the U.S.-Mexico border area that sought to improve the health of communities, using a community development approach as described by Rothman (1970). The methods used to organize the community and an immunization program designed by community health promoters will be described, and the mistakes made by the project staff in the planning phase will be discussed.

Project Description

The cities of northern Mexico along the border with the United States have public health problems similar to those in other areas of Mexico. However, because of their location far from Mexico City and close to the United States, they also suffer unique administrative, political, and health care-related difficulties (see Chapter 6 of this book). The proximity to the United States and the growth of the twin plant (*maquiladora*) industry have led to an increase in in-migration from the interior of Mexico. The twin plants, or *maquilas,* are owned by companies in the United States, Japan, and other countries. An agreement made in 1965 between the United States and Mexico allows these plants to exist in Mexico and to hire Mexican workers at the Mexican minimum wage, which in 1988 was less than $4 U.S. per day. The promise of jobs, either in the twin plants or in the United States, entices the poor to move to the cities on the border. The cities in this border area struggle to provide basic sanitation and health care to rapidly growing populations on a limited budget. Newcomers to the cities often live in small settlements (*colonias*) just beyond the reach of city services. Many of these *colonias* have no access to clean water, proper drainage, or electricity. According to the Ciudad (Cd.) Juárez Health Department (hereafter referred to as Salubridad), the major problems in these outlying *colonias* include preventable communicable diseases, especially waterborne diseases, controllable chronic diseases such as diabetes mellitus and hypertension, preventable accidents, and underimmunization of children less than 5 years of age.

In response to these problems in the Cd. Juárez, Chihuahua, and El Paso, Texas, border area, Project Verdad was formed as a joint effort of the National Presbyterian Church of Mexico and the Presbyterian Church (USA). Using methods of community development, the project addressed issues of education, economic development, church development, and health. The following sections will describe the health activities of the project.

The Health Program

In planning the health program, the PRECEDE planning model (Green & Kreuter, 1980; also see Green & Kreuter, 1991, for an updated version of this model) was employed. The PRECEDE model suggests that planners "begin at the end" by first engaging in a social diagnosis. In this first phase of planning, the planner and the community together determine the quality-of-life indicators for the community, the perceived needs of the community, and the goals of the community for the common good. Later phases involve the epidemiological diagnosis, in which health problems are defined; the behavioral and environmental diagnosis, in which links between behavior and health problems and the environment and health problems are assessed; and the educational and organizational diagnosis, in which predisposing, reinforcing, and enabling factors are assessed. *Predisposing* factors are antecedents to behavior that give the motivation to behavior, including knowledge, beliefs, values, and attitudes; *enabling* factors are antecedents to behavior that allow the person to act, such as availability of resources, access to health care, policies, laws, and community commitment; and *reinforcing* factors are things that occur after a behavior that provide a reward and encourage the continuation of the behavior.

The social and epidemiological diagnoses were completed by project staff along with community members already involved in other aspects of the project. Community meetings, focus groups, discussions with key informants, meetings with health officials, and door-to-door surveys were used to assess the needs of the community. The behavioral diagnosis was done in much the same way. For each behavior linked to health problems, the predisposing, reinforcing, and enabling factors were named and addressed in planned interventions. Many of the health problems on the border are not specifically related to behavior, but rather related to social and environmental problems that are difficult to address. The goal of the project was not only to change health behavior but to empower communities to attempt social and environmental change through community organization. Because Project Verdad was a church project, not related to a government organization or agency, it was easier for us (though not easy by any means) to organize communities around political issues. For the public health professional working with a government agency, this can be very difficult, especially if the goals of the community are not in accordance with the goals of the agency. Even more difficult is the situation in which the agency for which one works is the target of the community's ire. These are some of the most difficult issues that a health worker can face. The employee must decide how to deal with the tension between what the community wants and needs and what the agency wants and needs (see Minkler, 1978, for more on this issue).

Project Verdad staff also had the luxury of having time to "hang out" with the community. This is usually impossible for the health educator, nurse, or social worker, who must accomplish many tasks in a short period of time. Still, it is essential to get to know the community as much as possible. In many cases, agencies have found that community volunteers are willing to act as liaisons between the agency and the community and can give important feedback about needs and possible solutions.

The Project Verdad health program involved provision of primary care services, health education, and health promoter training. The health team included a U.S. health educator, two Mexican physicians, seven Mexican Presbyterian ministers, and one U.S. Presbyterian minister. An effort was made to involve the community in every aspect of the program. Mexican government health agencies were also included in planning and were essential advocates in many programs. Coalitions of community members and health and welfare agencies were formed on both sides of the border to encourage joint problem solving.

Community Development

Although we had hoped to use what we considered a "pure" locality development approach, in which all of the ideas about needs and all solutions sprang from the community itself, we often found that communities were unable to see how serious some health problems might be. The compromise was to insist on the maximum amount of community involvement but to "push" certain issues that were clearly important to the health of the residents. The community's "felt needs" were also discussed, prioritized, and addressed as much as possible. This seemed to be the best possible blend of locality development and social planning.

Primary Care

All seven Mexican communities and both U.S. communities with which we were involved felt the need for primary care services. Because many of the *colonia* residents were not insured by the Mexican social security program, they had few options for care. The primary care clinics were started by the project years before the full health program was considered and were continued as an important link with the community. The clinics provided basic sick care, immunizations and well-child care, well-woman care, and health education. Community volunteers assisted in the clinics, and communities helped in the maintenance and upkeep of the clinic sites. Primary care services were provided by one full-time Mexican physician, who also assisted with health promoter training and community development as part of the health promotion team, and one part-time Mexican physician, who also served as a part-time pastor for one of the small churches.

Health Education

Health education was provided at first by project staff and later by community health promoters. The focus of much of this education was on prevention and treatment of diarrhea and dehydration; prevention and treatment of common communicable diseases such as hepatitis A, strep infection, amebiasis, and scabies; and family planning. School health education was provided to the children in the project kindergartens and occasionally to public schools and public school teachers.

Health Promoter Training

One of the most important parts of the health program was the training of community health promoters because community "insiders" are better able to discover needs, relate to community values, and communicate health information than people from outside the community. The health promoters acted not only as respected teachers in the communities but as role models for their peers. Before the training program was started, community meetings were held to discuss problems and prioritize community concerns. Many of the *colonia* residents were interested in learning more about health and were especially concerned about child health problems. It was important to find individuals who were respected and trusted by the community. Health promoters were selected in two ways. First, we went to community leaders and key informants and asked about residents who might want to be trained and whom people in the community would know and trust. These promoters were recruited directly. Second, we offered basic health classes to anyone in the community. Those attending the classes who showed an interest in community involvement and who seemed to have the respect of their peers were recruited to be health promoters. Respect of peers was assessed in casual conversations with individual students and by taking note of whom others in the classes looked to for advice during class sessions. The health promoters were trained in basic health care, sanitation, and public health education methods. Their main focus was on issues seen as problems by both the communities and the health officials. These were family planning, immunizations, and diarrhea and dehydration prevention and treatment. Later projects involved water treatment programs and community health fairs.

Over a 2-year period, project staff recruited and trained approximately 40 adult women as health promoters (as well as 20 older children who were trained in care of younger siblings). Enthusiasm was high at first, following the graduation ceremony and presentation of equipment (thermometer, stethoscope, blood pressure cuff, first aid supplies). Within several months, however, we were left with a core group of about 15 women. Others had underestimated the amount of time that community work would involve, had taken jobs in the twin plants (we were unable to pay the health promoters), or had lost interest. The 15 remaining adult health promoters were of slightly higher educational level, were older on average, and felt that community service was a very important aspect of their lives.

Project Verdad's vision was that the health promoter training program would span a 6-year period. By the end of that time, it was expected that the health promoters would be on their own and working in coordination with health agencies to address public health problems in their *colonias.* Unfortunately, because of political and theological differences between the two churches (which were unrelated to the health project), the program was halted after only two and one-half years. During the 6 months following closure, the project staff made efforts (which were only partly successful) to tie the health promoters into another system. Despite these difficulties, there were many successful programs, including drinking water safety, health fairs, family planning, and immunization projects. The following is a summary of one of the more successful projects undertaken by the community health promoters during the last year of the program.

The Immunization Project

One of the most successful projects was developed by a group of three health promoters from one of the Cd. Juárez *colonias* for a neighboring community. They had been part of the original group of health promoters trained and had continued as active health promoters in their own *colonia.*

The health promoters were concerned for the children of this nearby community, which was located in the city dump only one street away from the health promoters' *colonia.* The health promoters considered the dump residents neighbors very similar to themselves but a bit poorer. One of the health promoters, because of the small grocery store run by her family, was well acquainted with many people in this community (this store was part of the project's economic development program). Most residents made their living picking usable items out of the garbage and repairing or making them into something they might sell. About 150 families lived in the area.

The first step taken by the health promoters was to survey the community. In a door-to-door survey it was discovered that approximately 50% of the community children were underimmunized or not immunized at all. The timing of this survey was of great importance in the health promoters' decision to begin an immunization program because it was done in the midst of a measles outbreak in the cities of Cd. Juárez and El Paso.

In casual discussions with women in the neighborhood, the health promoters discovered that there were several determinants of the lack of immunization coverage. First, the nearest health clinic was not within walking distance, and many of the mothers did not want to spend the day on the bus to get to the clinic. Second, because most of the residents were self-employed, they were not covered by the social security health plan (the social security plan, IMSS, provides medical coverage to most Mexican workers; see Chapter 6 of this book). Third, many of the babies and young children had never been officially registered, and many residents reported that most clinics would not immunize a child without a birth certificate. Although there had been several immunization campaigns in the area, many of the families had not participated, and those who had were unsure of the kind of vaccine received.

The health promoters decided that their goal would be to increase the number of fully immunized children in the area. After discussions with the community residents, they decided on the following plan of action:

1. Hold a monthly immunization clinic within walking distance of the *colonia,* run by the same health promoters every month.

2. Canvass the community monthly to advertise the clinic date and to answer questions about immunizations.

3. Provide record cards for keeping track of immunizations to those residents without the official card received on registration of birth, and encourage families to register children.

The first site chosen for the clinic was the small Presbyterian church located near the dump. After two clinics were held there, the health promoters decided to move the clinic to the grocery store site. Attendance improved dramatically when the site was changed, probably because the largely Catholic population was afraid that attempts would be made to convert them to Protestantism. Although the health promoters (many of whom were not Presbyterian) did not try to coerce community members to join the Presbyterian church, this was a valid concern because other "evangelical" Protestant groups were known for this behavior. A small living room in the back of the store for the use of the family during slow times was employed as the clinic. The health promoters kept records of the children attending the clinics and reported to Salubridad the number of immunizations given on a monthly basis.

The vaccine was made available to the project physicians by Salubridad. They were very cooperative and happy to have assistance in the campaign to immunize all the children of Juárez. A refrigerator located at a project clinic in a nearby *colonia* was set aside for vaccines. Another community health promoter who lived in this *colonia* was responsible for checking the temperature daily and maintaining the cold chain. On the day of the immunization clinic, vaccines were transported from this site to the grocery store in an ice chest.

During the first 2 months at the grocery store, the health promoters immunized approximately 50 children per month. The number decreased to about 20 per month in the third month of the program because more children were fully immunized and did not need to return. By the fifth month, about half of the children were returning to receive a follow-up vaccination.

Residents commented that they liked having a clinic within walking distance. Because the two health promoters who canvassed the community and gave immunizations every month were very similar to the *colonia* residents but a bit better educated and of a slightly higher socioeconomic status, they were trusted by the community and were considered appropriate reference persons (Suls & Miller, 1977). The health promoters also provided important modeling in that they had their children immunized at the clinic. Social reinforcement in the form of praise for the behavior of immunizing children was provided by the health promoters, the local pastor (who also encouraged his church members to attend), and other project staff. Modeling by similar others and social reinforcement are considered important determinants of behavior change (Bandura, 1986).

With the loss of the project, the health promoters were unable to continue the immunization clinic. An overseeing physician was required to obtain the vaccine, and project staff were unable to find a physician willing to take on this responsibility. Physicians were uncomfortable with signing for vaccine to be used by health promoters in whose training they had not participated and who were not known to them.

Discussion

Community organizing methods are helpful in empowering communities to solve problems. Because communities are not always aware of problems and may need the input of outside experts, the locality development approach and the social planning approach can be used jointly. Outside experts can assist the community in identifying and prioritizing problems, with the goal of working through the process so that in the future they will be able to repeat it on their own. Often the felt needs of the community are very different from the needs perceived by the outsider, and this must be carefully considered. The members of the community, after all, know more about themselves than the outsider. On the other hand, the outsider may have information that is not available to communities about particular problems. It is important, then, to share information and reach consensus about priority problems. If the community members are actively involved in this process, they will be more likely to feel ownership of the program and to continue working together.

Once problems have been identified, it is important to understand the determinants of the behavior. Members of the community are often the best investigators. Because others in the community will be more likely to trust them, informal community leaders can be very helpful in researching determinants of behavior. Focus groups and community meetings also give insight into the reasons people behave in certain ways. In planning interventions, community members must be involved because they will know what will be accepted and what will be rejected on the basis of the values, beliefs, and past experiences of the community (Rogers, 1983). Community health promoters can be trained to look for important predisposing, enabling, and reinforcing factors and to consider these factors when planning interventions.

Once the community program is in place, the community should carefully monitor the program. If they find that something is not working, they can plan together to change the approach. For example, when the church did not appear to be the best place to have the clinic, the health promoters took the time to discover why this was the case and were able to find a solution that was acceptable to them and the community. These monitoring and decision-making skills should be part of any community development program because the idea is to leave behind a community able to work through its own problems.

There are many ways that Project Verdad could have improved the chances of the health program continuing. The following are suggestions that might have improved the chances of program success.

1. The health promoters should have owned more of the program. For instance, perhaps they should have been responsible for making the arrangements with Salubridad and finding a physician willing to work with them. Instead, the project physician made contact with Salubridad, and the health promoters never met the most influential participants in that agency. We recommend that health professionals step back and allow community members to do as much of the planning and implementation as possible.

2. The health promoters should have been better connected to the Mexican government agencies involved in health promotion. A smoother transition might have been ensured if the health promoters had already been a part of the larger system. Although this involvement with existing agencies was in the project plans, it was not begun from the very start because it was somehow "easier" for the staff to make these connections. This linkage approach (Orlandi, Landers, Weston, & Haley, 1990), in which the target group is highly involved in all aspects of program planning, is a very important part of the community development process.

3. No plans had been made for compensation to the health promoters. Besides a certificate of course completion and a bag with a sphygmomanometer, a stethoscope, a thermometer, and first aid supplies, the health promoters received no compensation for their work. The project suffered considerable loss of health promoters even before the project closure, in part because women in the communities needed to help support their families. A system in which communities would find a way of reimbursing health promoters for their work would ensure lower attrition.

4. In general, the idea behind community development is for professional health workers to "work themselves out of a job." In other words, the community should be empowered to continue their work without outside interference. Structures must be put into place as the project is being planned to allow for this. As communities begin to work with professionals to plan health projects, they should be encouraged to take the lead in

contacting agencies and involving them in the program. It is not useful to wait until the program is established to make these connections because circumstances beyond the community's control may end the professionals' involvement sooner than expected.

Project Verdad sought to improve the health of communities using community development methods. Although some very successful programs were developed, the sudden, unexpected death of the project ended many of them. It is important to involve the community from the very beginning, not only in project planning and implementation but also in planning for such eventualities.

References

Alinsky, S. (1972). *Rules for radicals: A pragmatic primer for realistic radicals.* New York: Vintage.

Bandura, A. (1986). *Social foundations of thought and action.* White Cliffs, NJ: Prentice Hall.

Freire, P. (1970). *Pedagogy of the oppressed.* New York: Seabury.

Green, L., & Kreuter, M. (1980). *Health education planning: A diagnostic approach.* Palo Alto, CA: Mayfield.

Green, L., & Kreuter, M. (1991). *Health education planning: An educational and environmental approach.* Mountain View, CA: Mayfield.

Minkler, M. (1978). Ethical issues in community organization. *Health Education Monographs, 6,* 198-210.

Minkler, M. (1992). Community organizing among the elderly poor in the United States: A case study. *International Journal of Health Services, 22,* 303-316.

Nyswander, D. (1967). The open society: Its implications for health educators. *Health Education Monographs, 1*(22), 1-13.

Orlandi, M., Landers, C., Weston, R., & Haley, N. (1990). Diffusion of health promotion innovations. In K. Glanz, M. Lewis, & B. Rimer (Eds.), *Health behavior and health education.* San Francisco: Jossey-Bass.

Rogers, E. (1983). *Diffusion of innovations.* New York: Free Press.

Rothman, J. (1970). Three models of community organization practice. In F. M. Cox (Ed.), *Strategies of community organization: A book of readings.* Itasca, IL: F. E. Peacock.

Suls, J., & Miller, R. (1977). *Social comparison processes.* New York: Hemisphere.

Chapter 13

⚜

HEALTH OUTREACH PROGRAMS IN THE *COLONIAS* OF THE U.S.-MEXICO BORDER

JESUSA LARA

The influx of immigrants from Mexico has created a number of communities along the U.S.-Mexico border that are isolated from mainstream society for various reasons and are known as *colonias*. These *colonias* are usually without the benefits of water, sewage, and construction standards and are further handicapped by poor environmental sanitation and no ready access to basic health care services.

The Project Communities

Many *colonias* abound in El Paso County, located just across from Ciudad Juárez, Chihuahua, Mexico. Three communities, each composed of a number of *colonias*—namely, San Elizario, Montana Vista, and Canutillo—were the sites for the School Centered Health Education and Services for Rural Communities project in September 1990. The project was

AUTHOR'S NOTE: This chapter is based on the project School Centered Health Education and Services for Rural Communities, conducted by the College of Nursing and Health Sciences of the University of Texas at El Paso. The project was supported by a grant from the W. K. Kellogg Foundation. I have also written an article based on this project that was published in *Family and Community Health* (July 1994) and presented at a panel at the 1994 American Nurses Association Biennial Convention in San Antonio.

funded by the W. K. Kellogg Foundation for 3 years, from September 1990 to November 1993.

At the start of the project, San Elizario was a low-income community of approximately 3,500 people about 30 miles from El Paso. There was no public transportation. The lack of a sewage system and the use of individual wells in a high-water-table area increased the need for health promotion and disease prevention strategies. The community had many health care needs but very few services.

Some of the health problems that concerned the people were dental disease, hepatitis A, diabetes, hypertension, obesity, and drug abuse (Nickey, 1989; Sawyer & Brown, 1988). The community had only one full-time health worker, the school nurse. The local health department provided only an immunization and diabetes clinic once a month.

Montana Vista is another community with similar health problems to San Elizario. It is located 25 miles from downtown El Paso. There were about 800 families in 1990, with 1,500 children in school. (Population estimate now is about 15,000.) There was also no public transportation and no safe drinking water, and the only health care provider was the school nurse on school days.

Canutillo is also a medically underserved community outside El Paso. It is, however, closer to the city (approximately 12 miles), and the city/ county health district maintains a clinic there twice a week. Compared to the other two communities, it is considered superior in terms of the care available. To maximize the resources of the Kellogg grant, Canutillo was not included in the health services delivery portion of the project, but it shared in the health career promotion and health education activities.

Project Goals

A major goal of the project was to promote health careers as a long-term solution to the acute shortage of professional health care providers in these areas. It was hoped that some of the students exposed to health careers would eventually become health professionals and go back to serve their community. Strategies to meet this goal that were undertaken in school settings included health education classes, orientation of school children to health careers, role modeling by nursing students, holding of health career days, field trips to the College of Nursing and Health Sciences, and organization of health clubs in the schools. Essay, poster, and collage contests on health-related topics were also conducted to enhance awareness and promote interest in health careers.

To determine the effectiveness of these activities, participants were asked to fill out evaluation questionnaires at the end of each activity. School nurses, teachers, counselors, and nursing students involved in the program were also asked to evaluate the activities. Student nurses who conducted various activities used monitoring tools that included a student questionnaire, a health club activities summary, and a student weekly monitoring form.

The end goals of the project were provision of health education and primary health care services to the *colonia* residents. Two full-time registered nurses (RNs), who served as both community health nurse coordinators (CHNCs) and service providers, and nursing and allied health students were hired to carry out the activities. A seven-member advisory board, a nursing consultant, and the dean of the College of Nursing and Health Sciences (CNHS) provided guidance.

Strategies Used to Access the Community

At the onset of the project, several strategies were used to facilitate active participation by the Mexican American residents in the project sites. First, to promote trust and ready access, community schools were used as settings for disseminating information about the project. The schools are the "authority" in these communities, where there is rarely any other public service agency. Through the schools, the project staff were introduced to the community during school board and parent-teacher organization meetings.

A health education center known as Centro Educacional de Salud (CEDS) was established in each community, managed by a CHNC. The CEDS served as both a clinic and a multipurpose center for many activities in the community, there being no other place where people could congregate.

Initially, the project staff conducted a survey of the residents to find out if they were aware of the various career options in the health field and if they desired health careers for their children. Sixty percent of those who responded to the survey considered health careers for their children. The three professions most desired by the respondents for their children were nursing, medicine, and dentistry. Only a few respondents were aware of other health career options.

The residents were also asked about their perceptions of the needs and problems of the community. The survey revealed their priority needs to be dental service, immunization, health screening (blood pressure, vision, hearing), emergency medical service (EMS), a diabetic clinic, and family planning. The information gathered from this survey guided the planning and implementation of project activities.

Private and government health agencies willingly extended their services to these underserved areas through the CEDS on the request of the CHNC. Thus, health education classes and basic health and social services were provided at the CEDS, including immunization, blood pressure screening and monitoring, well-baby clinics, diabetic screening, and adult health clinics, by project staff, students, and other professional health care providers. Community meetings, exercise classes, and Alcoholics Anonymous meetings were also held there. A representative from the Department of Health and Human Services (DHHS) made weekly visits to facilitate residents' access to health and social services. Project staff also referred clients to appropriate agencies. Nursing students and staff visited clients in their homes. As more and more health and social services were coordinated by the project staff and provided to the residents, the latter developed a greater interest in participating in the planning and implementation of various health activities.

Training of Volunteer Community Health Workers (VCHWs)

Adults in the community were invited to participate in a VCHWs' training program to prepare them to assume a more active role in meeting the health needs of their families, friends, and neighbors. Topics discussed included team building, community organization, basic health assessment, management of simple home emergencies, parenting, nutrition, and environmental sanitation. Teaching was done by project staff, students, and other health care professionals recruited by the CHNC. The curriculum was written by the project staff on the basis of the communities' needs and problems. A total of 94 volunteers from the three project sites finished the VCHWs' course.

As VCHWs, they helped register clients in the clinics; took vital signs, heights, and weights; and monitored blood pressures. They also conducted home visits, door-to-door screening for diabetes, and a great deal of community health education. Home visits and house-to-house campaigns by nursing students, project staff, and VCHWs proved to be an effective strategy for mobilizing optimal community participation. Face-to-face meetings with the people in their own homes conveyed sincere interest in their health concerns and respect for their ideas as well as the worth of their individual contributions. Residents who initially declined telephone invitations to attend community meetings were persuaded to participate after being visited at home.

Initially, most of the *colonia* residents were not receptive to the idea of accepting responsibility for their own health care. They viewed the health professionals as the experts, whose job was to take care of lay people's health. Gradually, however, through continuous health teaching in the home and at the CEDS, lectures in the schools, and one-on-one discussions with the residents at every opportunity, project staff engendered the idea of taking responsibility for one's own health to the community. The VCHWs in one community were instrumental in organizing the residents to form an association that was officially incorporated and specifically delegated to work for the continuance and expansion of the health care services provided by the project. Primarily because of the work of this association, this community (Montana Vista) was awarded a multipurpose building by the Center for Housing and Urban Development of Texas A&M University, thus providing also a place for other health care providers.

Another goal of the project was to contribute to the knowledge base on effective strategies for meeting the health needs of rural Mexican Americans. Lessons learned from the training of the VCHWs and their involvement with community activities met this goal. The VCHWs became more politically involved in upgrading their communities. They identified some health needs and problems they wished to address, such as unsafe drinking water, transportation, poor sanitation, and youth-related problems, at the end of the project. Since then, they have made some progress in the solution of some of these problems.

Lessons Learned

To mobilize the communities to participate in the health activities, certain strategies were noted to be quite effective:

- The VCHWs proved to be the most effective agents for community mobilization. They got across information to the community regarding the project, recruited people to attend meetings and participate in activities, and facilitated community assessment and organization.
- Time and effort devoted to building awareness of and understanding of the role of the project, other health agencies, and the community residents in the improvement of the community's health situation also proved very helpful.
- Frequent home visits by health professionals facilitated the development of trust and encouraged more positive responses to health issues.

On the other hand, some cultural and religious beliefs and practices, inability to speak English, lack of transportation, and lack of family support were observed to slow down the mobilization process. More than 90% of the population in these communities spoke and understood only Spanish. This limited their participation in some activities because not all health care providers spoke Spanish and many health information materials were available only in English. The project staff did try to use both Spanish and English in all project activities.

Some beliefs, such as acceptance of certain illnesses as a matter of chance or a punishment from God (*castigo de Diós*), also prevented people from seeking treatment or participating in disease-preventive or health-promotive activities. Another factor was the residents' time orientation, which was relative. Strict attention was not given to the exact time of days for appointments; hence, health classes and meetings were often delayed, slowing down the mobilization process. Last, the lack of transportation, speedy means of communication, and family support (e.g., usually no relatives or close friends) also deterred residents from participating fully in community endeavors.

Recommendations

This Kellogg-funded project used the World Health Organization primary health care concept of self-reliance in the delivery of culturally sensitive health care to *colonia* residents in southwest Texas along the Texas-Mexico border (Lara, 1994). To gain the support and participation of the residents, the community was involved at the start and made to feel "genuine ownership" of the project. This also ensured continuity of community involvement in improving health care beyond the project period. The use of trained VCHWs as the main agents for mobilizing community participation facilitated achievement of project goals with very valuable outcomes for the community and is highly recommended. In border states where Hispanics have become the emergent majority, strategies to overcome language, cultural, and religious barriers must be given priority in the planning and implementation of any health care program.

References

Lara, J. (1994). Testing strategies for community participation and mobilization in health care. *Family and Community Health, 17,* 80-82.

Nickey, L. (1989). Health along the United States-Mexico border. *El Paso Physician, 8,* 8.

Sawyer, J., & Brown, J. (1988). *San Elizario health survey: Final report.* Unpublished manuscript.

Chapter 14

⎯∽⊱∽⎯

DIVINE RESOURCES

Health Education Activities at Churches Along the U.S.-Mexico Border

MICHAEL P. KELLY

Several studies indicate that religiosity is related to health behaviors and attitudes (Ferraro & Albrecht-Jensen, 1991; Kelly & Colwell, 1996; King, 1990; Ruppel, 1969; Wise, 1942; Woodroof, 1985). Ferraro and Albrecht-Jensen (1991) stated that people who pray and actively participate in their religion have better health, but those of a conservative religious affiliation are likely to be associated with poorer health status. Woodroof (1985) found religious behavior to be an important correlate to sexual behavior. Health educators, community health nurses, and other health and health care professionals are constantly searching for new channels to reach individuals with important health messages and services. Places of worship are logical and potentially effective locations for delivery of health education and services in the U.S.-Mexico border region.

Health and the religious experience are unique to humans. Certainly animals and plants can become diseased, injured, and die. Only humans, however, possess a spiritual element that makes a comprehensive model of health possible (Hoyman, 1966). Bensley (1991) concluded that some professionals define spiritual health in relation to the sense of fulfillment in life, whereas others concentrate on values and beliefs of community and self. Spiritual health may also be defined as a component of wholeness in life, spiritual wholeness, and spiritual well-being. In addition, the spiritual dimension may be defined in terms of a controlling higher power, a "godlike" force, and the human/spiritual interaction (Bensley, 1991).

Humans ask the tough questions: "Where did I come from?" "Why am I here?" and "Where am I going?" Religion frequently yields answers to these uniquely human questions, guides the formation of a value system, and provides a means to a healthy life and road to self-actualization. Humans long for meaning and solutions to life problems rather than just for pleasure or the avoidance of pain (Frankl, 1963). Everyone needs something to live for and live by because life is a marathon race, not a hundred-yard dash (Hoyman, 1966). A struggle for self-actualization without strong and clear values is absurd; one can only actualize to the extent to which one is fulfilling life's meaning. We all need something for which we would die, for only then do we possess something for which to live. Strong and clear values provide one with guidance in life. Pursuit of these values and life's meaning is the core of personal health, even for individuals struggling for life's most basic needs. In the pursuit of strong values, health, riches, and happiness may be found. The church can serve as an agent in formation, clarification, and strengthening of values, making clear that indeed man does not live by bread alone.

Because religion is fundamentally a means through which individuals and groups seek a way of life leading to a solution to life problems, and because health and illness are definitely the result of the kind of solution reached, religion, illness, and health are inextricably related at the very center as well as on the periphery of life. The symbols and techniques of religion, therefore, may be used to foster and reinforce unhealthy tendencies either in individuals or in cultures, or they may be used to change either individuals or cultures in the direction of health (Wise, 1942). In traditional cultures as well as in modern society, religion is a primary determinant of personal health.

Ancient and traditional cultures frequently attributed illness to angry deities, ancestral ghosts, or humans with supernatural powers. Despite personalistic causation or illness vectors, the root cause of the infirmity remains consistent throughout many traditional cultures. The root causes include loss of soul, object intrusion, spirit intrusion, disease sorcery, and breach of taboo. Although these root causes are categorically dismissed in modern society, cultural vocabulary still reflects traditional beliefs. A statement such as "They lost their will to live" derives from the soul loss theory of illness, and comments such as "I wonder what got into him" and

"I wonder what possessed him to do that" reflect concepts of spirit intrusion as a root cause of illness (Kinsley, 1996).

The paradigm of illness and health relating to religion is as ancient as religious healers. Many cultures relied on shamans, spirit mediums, priests, herbalists, and other holy persons for healing. Christian scripture records 41 cases of Jesus and the apostles healing the sick (Kinsley, 1996). Christians in modern cultures still submit names of the sick to their place of worship, pray for healing, practice faith healing, and request that religious leaders visit the sick. If history is any indication, religious establishments will continue to play a role in caring for the sick.

Tertiary disease treatment, secondary disease detection, and primary disease prevention can all be facilitated by religious organizations and, ideally, adopted as a primary mission of the church. The following discussion addresses tertiary, secondary, and primary health interventions as they relate to places of worship along the U.S.-Mexico border.

Tertiary health intervention typically occurs in a hospital, physician's office, or other clinical setting. The traditional role of religious organizations with respect to tertiary health intervention is providing spiritual and emotional comfort via pastoral visits to the sick as well as counseling. This limited paradigm is changing. Recent initiatives more frequently involve the church in expanded tertiary health intervention.

The Faith in Action program, supported by a national foundation, is one such initiative. This program, and others like it, helps organize people of all ages and faith groups to care for individuals with chronic health conditions within a community. Such programs draw attention to the needs of people with chronic health conditions and encourage the development of new community services to address them. This interfaith approach to tertiary care has yet to take hold in the border region.

Clergy perform important roles in healing the sick and at times serve as agents that further illness. The role of religious leaders in modern healing typically encompasses providing emotional support for the family and the sick and calling on divine intervention. Clergy frequently are appreciated for providing prayer, comforting words, and spiritual support. More psychological harm, however, can result from religious intervention if prayers, conversations, and personal actions emphasize death or a grave medical condition. Care must be taken, therefore, in planning pastoral visits to minimize the focus on the negative aspects of the medical condition so that the clergy do not become pathogenic agents themselves (Wise, 1942).

Health screenings, a form of secondary health intervention, can be an integral component of almost any planned health program. Mexican American women often seek medical attention at a more advanced stage of breast cancer than do non-Hispanics, often as a result of their failure to get or perform breast cancer screening (Vernon et al., 1992). This fact, combined with evidence that Mexican American women have higher rates of obesity, diabetes, and other disorders (Public Health Service, 1991), highlights the importance of health screenings at centers where Mexican Americans gather. Fitzhugh, Taylor, Vance, and Boll (1994) proposed the comprehensive health screening program planning model as one means of organizing health screenings. Previous research (Wells, Brown, Horm, Carleton, & Lasater, 1994) concluded that secondary health interventions, such as screening activities at churches, appeal to older members who reside near the place of worship. Furthermore, Davis et al. (1994) suggested that church-based screenings may be particularly valuable in providing access to underserved Hispanic women. This makes border churches a cost-effective contact point to screen for diabetes, cancer, and other diseases that disproportionately strike the elderly and Hispanics.

Sixteen million Americans have diabetes; half of these cases are undiagnosed, and over 3 million cases are diagnosed in adults age 65 and older. In addition, Mexican Americans represent 9.6% of diabetes cases; Cuban and Puerto Rican Americans represent another 20% (National Institute of Diabetes and Digestive and Kidney Disease [NIDDK], 1996). Considering that diabetes disproportionately affects the elderly and Hispanic population (NIDDK, 1996), places of worship along the U.S.-Mexico border are some of the most viable locations for secondary health intervention.

Screening activities at churches can be a prelude to primary health intervention. Research conducted by the University of Texas at El Paso and the El Paso Diabetes Association yields evidence that churches in the El Paso area are receptive to planned health screening activities. Of five churches approached in late 1995 and early 1996, all agreed to schedule diabetes screenings for their congregation. Though implementing screening activities on Sunday mornings can be logistically difficult, most parishioners in this El Paso study were supportive of health screenings, welcomed such initiatives, and patiently waited until they were screened. The screenings identified potential diabetics, provided a teachable moment at the church, and were useful for introducing parishioners to follow-up primary health intervention programs.

Support for primary health education interventions at places of worship is widespread (Kirn, 1991; Miller, 1987; Wilson, 1978; Wylie, 1996), and churches along the Texas-Mexico border are ideal places to implement health education programs. The church building may possess adequate physical space for instruction, educational equipment, and an effective communication system for all members. Religious organizations provide a natural gathering center and frequently have a multidisciplinary and talented membership with a long history of outreach and helping others (Lasater, Carleton, & Wells, 1991). Though churches are excellent resources for health intervention, the experienced health educator also promotes integration of health education into the church mission and fosters health promotion as a primary congregational mission. Viewing the church as only another resource or channel to be tapped in communitywide health education efforts is a limited model and may lead to unsuccessful programs.

Development of public/private partnerships in primary health education efforts is advocated by Broadbear (1995). Professionals in border health education should consider a partnership with places of worship. Be warned that bombarding a place of worship with a comprehensive health education program may not be wise. Starting with small initiatives—for example, promoting non-church-sponsored events, such as walk-a-thons— and achieving success is preferable to striving for an elaborate church-sponsored health education program and failing. On the other hand, easy success may lead to temporary programs; therefore, despite the size of the health promotion program, church members must have a feeling of program ownership and personal investment.

Constructs such as *fatalismo, machismo,* and *marianismo,* which stem from religion and culture, may influence health behaviors among Mexican Americans and must be anticipated when planning health promotion programs at places of worship. *Fatalismo,* the perception an individual can do little to prevent a disease or sickness, is common in Hispanic cultures (Carpenter, 1996). Combined with perceptions that illness is punishment from God, *fatalismo* hinders traditional health education techniques that rely on an internal locus of control and feelings of personal responsibility among participants. The macho demeanor, a social behavior pattern in which Latin males exhibit an overbearing attitude to anyone in a position they perceive as inferior to their own and demand complete subservience, is rooted in how God was perceived in Hispanic cultures (Wood & Price, 1997). *Marianismo,* the female complement to *machismo,* is also grounded in religion (Wood & Price, 1997). Health promotion programs at churches must recognize the constructs of *fatalismo, machismo,* and *marianismo* and allow for their expression and integration within planned interventions.

Just as churches employ a minister of finance, a minister of music, and a director of Christian education, there is room and need within churches for a minister of health. The minister of health may assist a senior clergy member, acting in a type of paraministry (Cafferky, 1982). Forming health programming committees, selecting and coordinating lay health advisors, organizing health resources, and communicating with community agencies capable of providing health services can be roles for the church health minister. In addition, the minister of health may select health education program models and assist in planning, implementing, and evaluating health programs. Irwin and Braithwaite (1997) stated that the church can be a valuable resource for healing, values, family and social support, client referrals, and community partnerships for health promotion. Their proposed four-phase comprehensive planning model for conducting health interventions in places of worship includes lay health workers from within the church as well as health professionals. The minister of health, as a professional trained in health promotion and education, may fill this need in a single congregation or coalition of churches.

In the mid-20th century, Wise (1942) stated that "training is absolutely essential for the student who hopes to discharge, to even a moderate degree, the responsibility which today is falling on the clergyman for the health and well-being of the community" (p. 264). Today, most health professionals still have little or no experience working with religious organizations (Lasater et al., 1991), and many ministers are inadequately trained to offer counsel in several health-related areas (Hyman, 1987). Despite lack of training, clergy are expected to provide care for infirm parishioners, and health educators are prompted to collaborate with places of worship in health promotion. In addition to training barriers, some other obstacles that serve to block health education efforts in religious settings are that the education may not be seen as appropriate, advantages for the religious organization may not be recognized, previous experience with health topics may not have been positive, suspicion and anxiety may develop about the impact on the organization's main mission, clerics may feel overly committed and fear new demands, and the organization may feel stressed and reluctant to take on new responsibilities (Lasater et al., 1991). Despite these barriers, the church remains a logical and potentially effective conduit for health information and a valuable provider of health promotion and education.

Planning health programs at places of worship is not vastly different from program planning for traditional communities. Differences, however, do exist. The following list contains specific suggestions for health professionals involved with church-based health interventions:

1. Incorporate prayer into planning and intervention activities. Christians frequently attribute illness to Satan or to humankind's fallen condition. This implies a low degree of individual responsibility for any given illness. The main personal responsibility, according to these interpretations, is to obtain the Lord's help in becoming healthy (McGuire & Kantor, 1988).

2. Begin programming at a slow rate, and, initially, plan events of easily manageable size. Achieve success in small doses, then gradually build larger programs on this success. An early success, however, may lead to a temporary program because the congregation forms little sense of ownership. The goal, then, is to help the congregation adopt health promotion as part of its mission and theological reason for being (Couture, 1993).

3. Incorporate health programming into existing functions. For example, when the church has a food-centered function, advocate the preparation of low-fat nutritious dishes.

4. Health programming will be more successful when working within the value and belief structure, as opposed to working against or attempting to circumvent it. For example, recognize the religion's stance on birth control, respect it, and design programs that honor parishioners' faith. Build on the overlapping value structure evidenced in religion and public health, recognizing the humanity of the church. The overlapping value structure includes caring for the poor, the oppressed, and the neglected (Couture, 1993).

5. Approach religious organizations as a system. Enlisting formal support from clerics, congregation officers, parishioners, and others involved in church is imperative for successful programming. Assist the faith group in forming a health programming committee, or incorporate the responsibility of health programming into an existing church committee.

6. Help the church develop and use models of health that include a spiritual, values-centered dimension. Use educational methods that help program participants identify and clarify personal values as well as the source of the values.

7. Be culturally sensitive, recognizing the multiplicity of Hispanic cultures. Accommodate individuals of varying degrees of acculturation, at times promoting acculturation as a means of community protection (Wood & Price, 1997).

8. Promote community ownership by empowering all Hispanic citizens, but especially females and families. Work within the confines of the *machismo*

and *marianismo* ethic, whenever possible harnessing elements that facilitate improved health status for Hispanics (Wood & Price, 1997).

Churches have a history of involvement with infirm parishioners. Programs such as Faith in Action build on this history of care for the sick. Though religious orientation may not directly determine the use of health care, it may still be a critical factor insofar as it contributes to the willingness of individuals to engage in certain health-related practices or hold certain health-related beliefs or attitudes that are causally antecedent to use (Schiller & Levin, 1988). Some churches are becoming more receptive to secondary health interventions such as diabetes and heart disease screening (Wells et al., 1994). Still more progressive churches are exploring the realm of primary health intervention, better known as health education and promotion (Davis et al., 1994). Considering the influence that churches have on citizens of the U.S.-Mexico border region, health professionals would be negligent to ignore this divine resource.

References

Bensley, R. (1991). Defining spiritual health: A review of the literature. *Journal of Health Education, 22,* 287-290.

Broadbear, J. (1995). The development of public/private partnerships and their impact on the future of public health. *Eta Sigma Gamma Monograph Series, 13*(1), 1-11.

Cafferky, M. (1982). Whole health education: The religious worker's role. *Journal of Health Education, 13*(2), 25-27.

Carpenter, V. (1996). Cancer knowledge, self-efficacy, and cancer screening behaviors among Mexican-American women. *Eta Sigma Gamma Monograph Series, 13*(1), 12-21.

Couture, P. (1993). *When public health and faith groups encounter each other* [On-line]. http://www.interaccess.com/ihpnet/couture

Davis, D., Bustamante, A., Brown, C., Wolde-Tsadik, G., Cheng, X., & Howland, L. (1994). The urban church and cancer control: A source of social influence in minority communities. *Public Health Reports, 109,* 500-506.

Ferraro, K., & Albrecht-Jensen, C. (1991). Does religion influence adult health? *Journal for the Scientific Study of Religion, 30,* 193-202.

Fitzhugh, E., Taylor, J., Vance, T., & Boll, A. (1994). Health screenings: A comprehensive program planning model. *Health Educator: Journal of Eta Sigma Gamma, 25*(2), 13-17.

Frankl, V. (1963). The significance of meaning for health. In D. Belgum (Ed.), *Religion and medicine* (pp. 177-185). Ames: Iowa State University Press.

Hoyman, H. S. (1966). The spiritual dimension of man's health in today's world. *Journal of School Health, 36*(2), 52-63.

Hyman, W. (1987). *Differential perceptions of ministers and churchgoers with regard to health counseling needs.* Unpublished doctoral dissertation, Texas A&M University.

Irwin, C., & Braithwaite, R. (1997). A church-based diabetes education program for older African-American women. *American Journal of Health Studies, 13*(1), 1-7.

Kelly, M., & Colwell, G. (1996). Condom embarrassment: Contributing factors. *Journal of Wellness Perspectives, 12*(2), 80-89.

King, D. (1990). Religion and health relationships: A review. *Journal of Religion and Health, 29*(2), 101-112.

Kinsley, D. (1996). *Health, healing, and religion: A cross-cultural perspective.* Englewood Cliffs, NJ: Prentice Hall.

Kirn, J. (1991). Religion and the health belief model. *Journal of Religion and Health, 30,* 321-329.

Lasater, T., Carleton, R., & Wells, B. (1991). Religious organizations and large-scale health related lifestyle changes programs. *Journal of Health Education, 22,* 233-239.

McGuire, M., & Kantor, D. (1988). *Ritual healing in suburban America.* New Brunswick, NJ: Rutgers University Press.

Miller, J. (1987). Wellness programs through the church: Available alternative for health education. *Health Values, 11*(5), 3-6.

National Institute of Diabetes and Digestive and Kidney Disease. (1996). *Prevalence of diabetes in the United States* [On-line]. http://www.niddk.nih.gov/ DiabetesStatistics/DiabetesStatistics.html

Public Health Service. (1991). *Healthy people 2000.* (DHHS Pub. No. 91-50213). Washington, DC: Government Printing Office.

Ruppel, H. (1969). Religiosity and premarital sexual permissiveness: A methodological note. *Sociological Analysis, 30,* 176-188.

Schiller, P., & Levin, J. (1988). Is there a religious factor in health care utilization? A review. *Social Science and Medicine, 27,* 1369-1379.

Vernon, S. W., Vogel, V. G., Halabi, S., Jackson, G. S., Lunday, R. O., & Peters, G. N. (1992). Breast cancer screening behaviors and attitudes in three racial/ethnic groups. *Cancer, 69*(1), 165-174.

Wells, B., Brown, C., Horm, J., Carleton, R., & Lasater, T. (1994). Who participates in cardiovascular disease risk factor screenings? Experience with a religious organization-based program. *American Journal of Public Health, 84,* 113-115.

Wilson, R. (1978). Religiosity and health: Implication for health promotion. *Health Values, 2,* 144-146.

Wise, C. (1942). *Religion in illness and health.* New York: Harper & Brothers.

Wood, M., & Price, P. (1997). Machismo and marianismo: Implications for HIV/AIDS risk reduction and education. *American Journal of Health Studies, 13,* 44-52.

Woodroof, J. (1985). Premarital sexual behavior and religious adolescents. *Journal for the Scientific Study of Religion, 24,* 343-366.

Wylie, W. (1996). A health education paradigm change encompassing religious settings. *Journal of Health Education, 27,* 122-125.

❦

Chapter 15

MIGRANT AND SEASONAL FARMWORKERS

Health Care Issues

SANDRA BENAVIDES-VAELLO
HEATHER SETZLER

A heterogeneous population of Black, White, Hispanic, Haitian and other ethnic backgrounds numbering between 2.7 and 5 million people, migrant and seasonal farmworkers endure substandard living conditions, labor in one of the most dangerous occupations in the nation, and have limited access to primary health care.

National Migrant Resource Program (1990a, p. 2)

This assessment of the conditions faced by the migrant and seasonal farmworker population, although accurate, merely scratches at the surface of the many aspects of the lives of these people without probing the profound challenges faced by farmworkers in the United States and those who attempt to provide care for them. Only by looking at the varied aspects of the migrant and seasonal farmworker population—who they are, where they live, and what problems they have—can one gain a fuller understanding of the needs of this population. More important, it is only with this understanding that one can more adequately assess how the health and wellness demands of the migrant and seasonal farmworker population can be realized.

Any inquiry to better understand the hardships endured by migrant farmworkers must first answer the difficult question regarding the composition of this population. Estimates of the number of migrant farmworkers in the United States generally range around 3 to 4 million, although there are estimates as low as 159,000 and as high as 5 million (K. Mountain, personal communication, September 15, 1993; Rust, 1990). The difficulty in enumerating the migrant population is due in part to the differences in definitions and ambiguity in the terms used for migrant farmworkers by those conducting surveys and releasing the results (Martin, 1988, p. 13). There is no standard definition for comparison across agencies (National Advisory Council on Migrant Health, 1992, p. 296). Further obstacles in determining the demographics of this population arise when one considers the large undocumented population, estimates of which vary from 20% to 60% of the total (K. Mountain, personal communication, September 15, 1993; R. Ryder, personal communication, September 10, 1993).[1] In general, what is known about the documented migrant farmworker population is that it is predominantly Hispanic, younger than average, largely a welfare population, and highly mobile (National Advisory Council on Migrant Health, 1993, p. 12).

The Special Agricultural Worker (SAW) and Replenishment Agricultural Worker (RAW) Programs enacted by the government in 1986 have also affected the numbers and composition of the migrant farmworker population. The SAW legalization program was part of the Immigration Control and Reform Act (IRCA) of 1986, which granted temporary residence status to agricultural workers who had done at least 90 days of qualifying agricultural work in the 12 months ending May 1, 1986. Applications were accepted between June 1, 1987, and November 30, 1988; during this time, 1.2 million workers applied for the benefits of this program. Of these, 350,000 were eligible to become "Group I SAWs," able to become permanent resident aliens after December 1, 1990 (Martin & Taylor, 1988).

Because the workers who applied for and received temporary residence status or permanent resident alien status through the SAW program were not obligated to remain in agricultural work, it was expected that many would choose to leave agriculture as an occupation. In anticipation of a shortage of agricultural workers, the Replenishment Agricultural Worker program was enacted in 1989. The RAW program issued visas similar to the temporary residence cards given to SAWs. After 3 years of farm work, RAWs are eligible to apply for permanent resident alien or green card status; however, RAWs can be deported if they do not work in seasonal agricultural services for at least 90 days out of every year (Martin & Taylor, 1988).

The migration patterns and mobility of the migrant farmworker population have led to the division of the workers in the United States into three different areas, or streams (see Figure 15.1). Each stream has its "home base" downstream, in a winter crop area, where the farmworkers base themselves for the majority of the year. From the home-base states, the farmworkers migrate upstream to harvest the seasonal crops of the "non-home-base" states. Often the workers, the majority of whom are married and/or have children, will migrate north to the non-home-base states while leaving their families in the home-base state for the season. The home-base states are Florida for the East Coast stream, Texas for the Midwest stream, and California for the West Coast stream. Due to the different migration influences as well as the differing crops, the demographics of the three U.S. streams have many differences.

Aside from the three streams in the United States, there are a significant number of migrant farmworkers who are home based in Mexico. Many of these farmworkers return home annually after the harvest season; others decide to migrate more permanently into the United States. The primary sending region in Mexico is the central plateau; about 70% of the migrants from Mexico to the United States come from the northern and western states of the central highlands (Mines & Massey, 1985). The states of Zacatecas, Michoacán, Jalísco, and San Luis Potosí are commonly cited as states from which many farmworkers migrate (Horton, 1989; Mines & Massey, 1985; Stoddard, 1984). Home bases have also been identified in the Mexican states of Coahuila and Chihuahua and in the communities of Ahuacatlan and Lacaja in the state of Guanajuato (N. Hook, personal communication, October 8, 1993; Horton, 1989).

In the East Coast stream, one finds a population that is primarily Puerto Rican, Haitian, and African American, with a strong and growing element of refugees from Latin America. In this group, the majority are single male workers; therefore, one will find a large number of camps along the East Coast that are designed for men without families (K. Mountain, personal communication, September 15, 1993).

The Midwest stream has a population that is over 95% Hispanic because many of the workers in this stream migrate directly into the stream from Mexico and south Texas. There is a larger prevalence of nuclear families

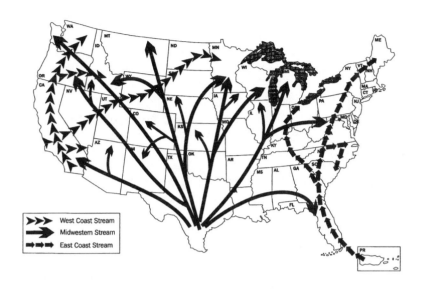

Figure 15.1. Major Migratory Streams for Farmworkers
SOURCE: National Center for Farmworker Health, Inc., Austin, TX. Reprinted with permission.

in this stream, and one therefore will encounter fewer gender-specific camps (K. Mountain, personal communication, September 15, 1993).

The West Coast farmers historically drew their workers from imported laborers—Chinese in the 1880s, Japanese in the 1900s, and southern Europeans and Filipinos into the 1930s—and then drew hordes of displaced Midwestern corn belt farmworkers during the Depression (Goldfarb, 1981, p. 11). Currently, however, the demographics of the West Coast stream indicate a sizable concentration of Hispanics, larger than that of the East Coast stream but not quite as concentrated as that of the Midwest. Generally, there has been a strong nuclear family presence in this stream as well as a number of single males. Recently, however, there has been an influx of single women, especially from Central America; hence, one currently is seeing some women-only camps, as well as the previously present men-only camps (K. Mountain, personal communication, September 15, 1993).

Determining the demographics of the migrant population as a whole and in each of the streams is a difficult task; it is even more challenging to ascertain the differing health problems and subsequent health demands of these populations. The Migrant Health Program (MHP; Section 329, Part D, Title III of the 1962 Public Health Service Act) finances migrant and community health clinics across the nation with federal funding equivalent to approximately $100 per user per year, so that they may provide the needed health care services to the migratory and seasonal farmworker population and their families (National Advisory Council on Migrant Health, 1993, p. 17). This program and others that will be discussed later in this chapter attempt to serve the migrant population but are not always successful in reaching the population in large enough numbers.

The prevailing health problems that are seen in the migrant health clinics are those of a disease cycle similar to that of the Third World or of the United States in the 1930s. Infectious, parasitic, and opportunistic diseases, such as tuberculosis, as well as other easily preventable health problems, such as malnutrition, are commonplace occurrences in the migrant health clinics (K. Mountain, personal communication, September 15, 1993). Up to 78% of the farmworker population suffers from parasitic infections at some time, compared with only 2% to 3% of the general population (NMRP, n.d.). A 1992 study in Florida found that 44% of the participants tested positive for tuberculosis (Centers for Disease Control and Prevention [CDC], 1992). The main reasons for the prevalence of these health problems are the housing and field conditions (i.e., poor sanitation and facilities) both at the home base and upstream, hunger, poverty, and the occupational hazards of agricultural work, such as exposure to pesticides and other dangerous substances and on-the-job injuries. Unfortunately, the occupational health and safety movement has been overwhelmingly oriented toward construction, manufacturing, and mining, even though agriculture is one of the most dangerous occupations (Sakala, 1987).

Health problems in this population are magnified and perpetuated by the difficulty of disease management due to the high mobility of migrant patients and lack of a viable data transfer system between clinics in different communities or states, as well as by the fact that the social services for the migrant farmworker population are poorly funded and inadequate (K. Mountain, personal communication, September 15, 1993). Federal funding under the MHP is granted to 105 migrant health centers nationwide. These funds are then distributed to approximately 400 clinic sites nationwide (see Figure 15.2), at which there are an estimated 500,000

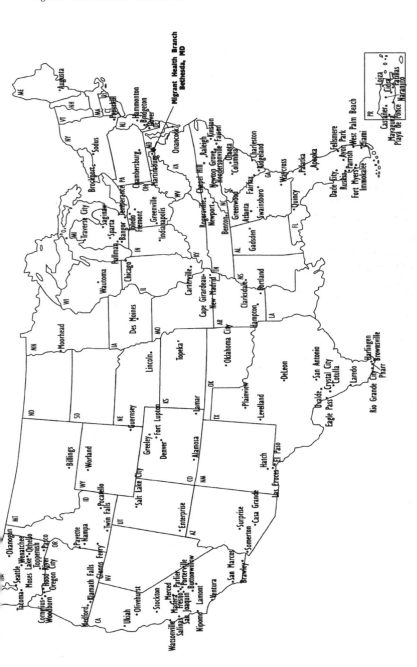

Figure 15.2. Migrant Health Centers Map
SOURCE: National Migrant Resource Program (1990b).

encounters per year (Rust, 1990; Wilk, 1986, p. 13). This accounts for approximately 13% of the migrant farmworker population. Most clinics that receive migrant health monies also receive funding through other federal programs and therefore provide services to other low-income families as well (National Association of Community Health Centers ([NACHC], 1991, p. 6). Except for Puerto Rico, there are no clinic sites in the United States that serve only migrants (A. Braña, personal communication, July 30, 1993).

A further concern is the low educational level of the farmworker population. The average educational level of migrant farmworkers was 6.4 years in a study conducted in 1986 (Littlefield & Stout, 1988). Without an adequate education, the concepts of health promotion and disease prevention are difficult to comprehend. This can have serious consequences for confronting a disease process such as AIDS. A 1988 study conducted in rural Georgia by Foulk, Lafferty, Ryan, and Robertson (1989) found that migrant farmworkers have lower levels of education about AIDS than the general population, leading to numerous false assumptions about the transmission of the disease and the disease itself. The need for the prevention of AIDS was not understood by 38.8% of the participants, who did not realize that AIDS is a fatal disease.

Just as the demographics and the agricultural influences change through the three streams, so do the prevalent health care problems. Furthermore, the health problems differ within each stream between the home-base and non-home-base states. In the home-base states, the border area is especially plagued with a multitude of problems. Given the poverty of the area and the inherent problems of two communities in close proximity with differing laws and health systems, the border area shows a higher incidence of infectious diseases and other health problems. Communicable diseases, such as hepatitis A, tuberculosis, and vaccine-preventable diseases such as measles, are more prevalent in border communities than in border states as a whole (Hatcher et al., 1995). These health issues are compounded by the poor housing conditions of the numerous border residents who live in *colonias*. *Colonias* are unincorporated settlements located on both the U.S. and Mexican sides of the border. These settlements are often devoid of running water, plumbing, electricity, sewer, and drainage systems (Warner, 1991). These circumstances provide a perfect medium for the perpetuation of disease transmission and poor health. Among the populations affected by these issues are migrant and seasonal farmworkers, many of whom live in these *colonias*.

Due to the time limitations of the research project—it was conducted as part of a year-long policy research project—and financial constraints that limited travel, the attention of the remainder of this chapter will be directed at Texas and the Midwest stream. The focus will be on the health status and access to health care of the population, and a summary of the general health conditions of this population will be followed by an overview of the available programs for migrant and seasonal farmworkers. Presentation and discussion of the results from the Health Care Accessibility Survey conducted in Webb and Cameron counties for this project and delineation of areas for further research will conclude the chapter.

General Health Conditions in the Midwest Stream

In 1986 and 1987, the Migrant Clinicians Network (MCN), with technical support from the National Migrant Resource Program (NMRP) and funding from the U.S. Department of Health and Human Services's Bureau of Health Care and Delivery Assistance and the MHP, examined data from four Midwest stream migrant health centers in Texas, Michigan, and Illinois, as well as from community health centers for two control group counties (Dever, 1991; see Appendix D of this book). The purpose of the study was to test the hypothesis that Hispanic migrant and seasonal farmworker populations differ from the Hispanic population per se. The findings of the study revealed that migrant farmworkers had age-specific health problems that are different and more complex than those of the general population. The farmworkers had more clinic visits than the general population for some health problems, including a higher-than-normal occurrence of infectious disease, diabetes, pregnancy, hypertension, and contact dermatitis and eczema. Their visits to the clinic for general medical exams, however, was 39% below the national average.

In general, the findings provide solid evidence that the health status of the farmworker population is far below that of the general population, as well as being different from that of other populations in terms of the problems it encompasses. Also revealed through this study was that the overall health of the home-base farmworkers, at least in the clinics studied, was significantly worse than that of the general U.S. population or farmworkers in non-home-base areas (Dever, 1991). Because the home-base states generally have a highly concentrated migrant and seasonal farmworker population, there is more competition for the available health services, leading to the disparity in the health status of the home-base versus non-home-base communities.

The high prevalence of infectious diseases in the farmworker population studied by the MCN is a serious issue because these diseases persist and progress amid the poor living conditions of the farmworker population. Among the concerns associated with substandard living conditions is water quality. In the summer of 1987, a community and migrant health center in Pullman, Michigan (Pullman Health Systems), conducted an assessment of the water quality of the wells serving the migrant and farmworker population. The results of these tests indicated that "some wells" were potential health hazards with either short- or long-term usage due to high levels of bacteria. The contaminant range in these wells was from 0 to 84 MF coliform count per 100 ml, whereas the safety limit for bacteria is 0 MF coliform count per 100 ml. This led the board of directors of the center to support a plan to test the wells annually in an effort to determine whether the nitrate concentration would increase from year to year. Future efforts of this center will focus on previous screening and education projects as well as the institutionalization of groundwater educational services (Miller, 1990).

Among the many problems suffered by both home-base and non-home-base migrant farmworkers in the MCN study, diabetes mellitus was the most common in the migrant health centers, accounting for 8.3% of the total diagnoses in the clinic during the study period (see Table 15.1) (Dever, 1991). The high incidence of gestational diabetes mellitus (GDM) was recognized by the certified nurse-midwives at the maternity center of the Brownsville Community Health Center in Texas, and this led to the development of a program of maternity care for gestational diabetes. This program tested the clients for GDM and then provided nutritional training and frequent testing for those diagnosed with it. The need for programs such as this one has been recognized in the Midwest Migrant Health Information Office (MMHIO). The Camp Health Aide Program was formulated by the MMHIO as an educational program designed to bridge the gap between the existing health care system and the health care needs of the migrant farmworkers. Migrant women (and a few men) are trained by MMHIO staff members to act as health resources in the migrant camps. This program, which began with a pilot program in Michigan in 1985 and has since expanded to eight sites in four Midwestern states, benefits farmworkers, health centers, outreach programs, and workers, as well as the participants themselves (Robinson, 1990). Although this program has been successful, a greater number of programs that facilitate the use of health services by the migrant farmworker population are needed.

Available Programs for Migrant and Seasonal Farmworkers

There are few health programs designated specifically for migrant and seasonal farmworkers. The federally funded MHP and the Gateway Community Health Center, Inc. Entitlement Program are two such programs. Medicaid covers those farmworkers who meet its eligibility requirements in each state, and there is currently a study being conducted to determine if an interstate reciprocity program would be feasible (Wright, 1993). In Texas, the Community Oriented Primary Care Association, Inc. (CO-PRIMA), although not exclusively for migrant and seasonal farmworkers, does provide services to eligible farmworkers (A. Gonzalez, personal communication, January 28, 1994).

Migrant Health Program

The MHP is a branch of the Division of Primary Care Services in the Department of Health and Human Services. A federally funded program created under sections 329 and 330 of the Public Health Service Act of 1964, the MHP served only migrant farmworkers from 1964 through 1970, when it was expanded to include services for seasonal farmworkers (Wright, 1993). The program is administered by the Health Resources and Services Administration (HRSA), and its budget for FY95 was $65 million, an 11.8% increase from FY94. The FY96 appropriations bill, which includes the funding for the Migrant Health Program, did not pass by the October 1 deadline; programs in this situation are currently being funded at a 5% reduction from FY95 levels (NACHC, 1996). Grants are distributed to health centers on the basis of the total number of migrant and seasonal farmworkers in their service area, with highest priority given to centers with over 6,000 migrant farmworkers and lowest priority given to those sites serving less than 6,000 seasonal agricultural laborers. Approximately 105 organizations, mostly nonprofit, receive direct funding, and then many distribute these funds to satellites or other centers (H. Kavenaugh, personal communication, April 19, 1994). Program eligibility is based on the family's preceding 2 years of employment in agriculture and income history.[2]

Gateway Entitlement Program

As of 1986, there were only a few farmworker hospitalization insurance plans nationwide, including Mutual of Omaha, Florida Agricultural Health Plan of Blue Cross/Blue Shield in Jacksonville, and the Gateway Community Health Center, Inc. Entitlement Program in Laredo. Of these, the Gateway Entitlement Program is the only one that continues to exist. It is a program funded by the U.S. Department of Health and Human Services in conjunction with Blue Cross/Blue Shield of Texas, Inc., which provides health benefits for enrolled migrant farmworkers. The total budget of the program is $345,000, which covers participants from Laredo for care in 49 counties in the Texas Panhandle and the rest of the United States for hospitalization and nonpreventive care (M. Treviño, personal communication, February 29, 1996).

Any farmworker home based in Webb County who does not have insurance coverage and can pay the registration fee (approximately $7.00/person) and monthly premium ($12.36/month/person) is eligible for coverage under this plan. Eight hundred and forty farmworkers and their dependents were covered in 1995-1996, a decrease from 938 in 1994-1995 and 1200 in 1993-1994.

COPRIMA

The Community Oriented Primary Care Association (COPRIMA) is a Texas Department of Health (TDH)-funded program that provides primary care coverage to eligible clients through contracts with local providers at 34 project sites in 76 Texas counties. Funding comes from the Community Oriented Primary Care Division of TDH. The total budget for the Brownsville site for FY96 is $345,712. To be eligible, one may not have any other type of insurance and must be employed. Proof of income, no more than 150% of the poverty level, state residency, photo identification, and the payment of a registration fee ($5.00/person below 100% poverty and $10.00/person above 100% poverty) are required for enrollment. Enrollees are covered for the period of 1 year unless there is a change in their eligibility. Coverage includes up to $100 each for emergency care and lab work or x-rays and $40 per month in medications and also provides health education classes in the *colonias*. The COPRIMA program in the city of Brownsville serves the four local *colonias* and currently serves around 825 clients, with a goal of 1,000 (A. Gonzalez, personal communication, March 8, 1996).

Health Care Accessibility Survey Results

Purpose

The purpose of the research was to investigate health care and health care accessibility problems faced by migrant and seasonal farmworkers. Because less than 15% of this population is being seen in the federally funded clinics and programs (NACHC, 1991), we were interested to find out whether the remainder were obtaining services in other U.S. facilities, in Mexico, or not at all. The sites of Brownsville and Laredo were chosen because south Texas serves as the home base for a significant number of migrant and seasonal farmworkers. A study of the farmworker population in Texas for 1987 estimated their numbers at 513,731 statewide. The 1987 estimates for the lower Rio Grande valley (including Cameron, Hidalgo, and Willacy counties) and the Laredo area (Webb County) are 265,807 and 12,568, respectively; these estimates combined represent 54.7% of the total estimated farmworker population in Texas (Plascencia, Ceballos, & Glover, 1989, pp. 74-79). The proximity of these two cities to Mexico was of further importance. The study was done in the late winter and early spring because at that time most workers have returned from their upstream work sites.

The *colonias* visited for the interviews, Rio Bravo in Laredo and Cameron Park and Olmito in Brownsville, house the majority of migrant and seasonal farmworkers in these two cities. Rio Bravo is an incorporated city located approximately 10 miles from Laredo and has a population of approximately 7,000. Cameron Park is about 3 miles from Brownsville and has a population of 4,000 to 5,000 inhabitants. Olmito is an incorporated city located approximately 5 miles north of Brownsville with 1,500 to 2,000 inhabitants (A. Gonzalez, personal communication, January 28, 1994; G. Peña, personal communication, December 3, 1993). The infrastructure in these *colonias* is poor. Inadequate street drainage and garbage collection have led to appalling and dangerous living conditions.

Methodology

The data collection tool used for the research was a survey with approximately 40 questions concerning demographics, housing conditions, migration patterns, health problems, and health care service utilization (see Appendix D). The survey was administered verbally in both Spanish and English to representatives of 47 migrant farmworker families. We conducted the survey interviews in the homes of the farmworkers and at clinic sites.

In Laredo, we contacted the Gateway Community Health Center, where Gloria Peña, Director of Patient Services, set up interviews with several migrant families at the clinic. Families who were visiting the Health Center for services were asked if they would be interested in participating in the research project. Those who agreed were interviewed at the clinic. Others interviewed in Laredo were identified by Lauro Garcia, Director of the Motivation, Education and Training Program in Laredo. In Brownsville, Tony Zavaleta, PhD, dean of the College of Liberal Arts at the University of Texas at Brownsville and director of COPRIMA, referred us to the administrative assistant of COPRIMA, Alice Gonzalez. A community worker with COPRIMA identified farmworker families in the *colonias* (Cameron Park and Olmito) outside Brownsville. She then asked their permission to be interviewed and accompanied us during the interviews.

Results

Demographics

Nearly all of the 47 migrant farmworkers interviewed were married (96%) and had children (89%). Seventy-seven percent of those responding to the survey were female. The average age of all respondents was 36.8 years, with ages ranging from 19 to 64. The average family had 3.5 children still living at home. The average age of the children living at home was 11.3 years, with ages ranging from 3 months to 32 years. Although 74% of the participants were born in Mexico, most stated that they were legal residents, and nearly all (98%) had resided in the United States for more than 5 years.

Housing Conditions

Eighty-five percent of those surveyed owned their own homes, although most were still making payments on the property; 13% rented; and

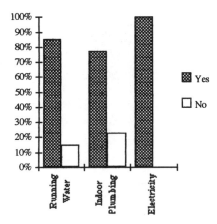

Figure 15.3. General Housing Necessities (*N* = 46)

2% (representing one family) had been unable to locate housing at the time of the interview. Basic housing necessities, such as running water and indoor plumbing, were lacking in a significant number of the houses of the farmworkers interviewed. Thirteen percent did not have running water, and 21% were without indoor plumbing (see Figure 15.3). Several of the participants were living in trailers and other recreational vehicles that had hookups; otherwise, it is not likely that most of these people would have had access to indoor plumbing and/or running water. There were an average number of six people living in homes with an average of two bedrooms (see Figure 15.4).

Migration Patterns

All participants maintained their home bases in Laredo and Brownsville, where most (87%) had lived for over 3 years. They migrated to numerous states for work. Twenty-two states were mentioned, with the most common being California, Florida, Michigan, Minnesota, and Ohio. Eighty-three percent had migrated annually for more than 3 years, and only a small percentage (6%) had entered the migrant stream in the past year. The importance of family unity during the migration was shown by the number of workers who traveled and worked with their spouse, children, and/or other extended family members (see Figure 15.5). Eighty-one percent traveled with their spouses, 81% with their children, and 49% with extended family members; only 6% traveled alone. Most of the families

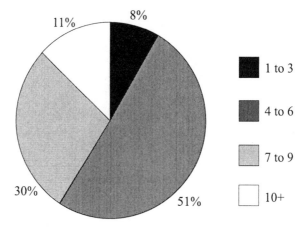

Figure 15.4. Number of Occupants per Household ($N = 47$)

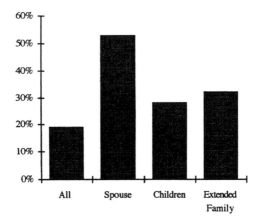

Figure 15.5. Migratory Labor Participants ($N = 47$)

lived and worked outside Texas for a period of 3 to 6 months annually (Figure 15.6). For many families, this migration occurred during the summer months, when the children were not in school and were able to work, indicating a strong education ethic and the vital role of the children's financial contributions to the families' survival.

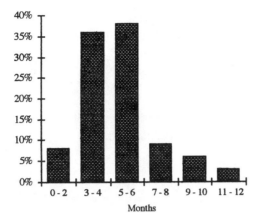

Figure 15.6. Duration of Yearly Migration (*N* = 47)

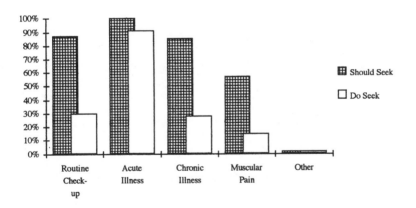

Figure 15.7. Medical Attention: Desired Versus Actual (*N* = 47)

Health Problems and Health
Care Service Utilization

Most respondents thought that one should seek medical attention under
various circumstances, including routine checkups, acute illnesses, chronic

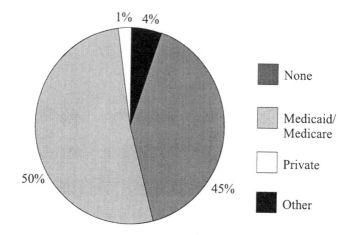

Figure 15.8a. Insurance Coverage: Children (*N* = 166)

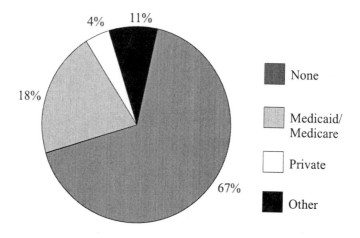

Figure 15.8b. Insurance Coverage: Adults (*N* = 92)

illnesses, and muscular pain or discomfort. However, the majority actually sought medical attention only when there was an acute illness (Figure 15.7). When asked what medical problems they had experienced in the past 2 years, 81% identified acute illnesses, such as ear infections and colds; only 36% had seen a health care provider for routine checkups. Considering

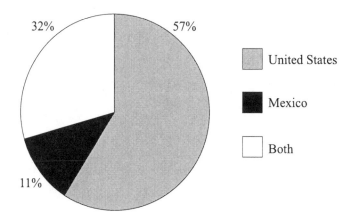

Figure 15.9. Binational Utilization of Health Care Services (*N* = 47)

the number of women interviewed, this indicates low participation in annual gynecological exams.

Although some families indicated that they were able to get insurance through their employment outside Texas, 67% of the adults and 45% of the children were uninsured at the time of the interviews. The largest insurer of children was Medicaid, at 49%, and 4% were covered through other agencies, including COPRIMA and the Gateway Entitlement Program (Figure 15.8).

Medical attention was sought in both the United States and Mexico. Fifty-seven percent of those interviewed used health care services exclusively in the United States, 32% used binational services, and 11% sought care only in Mexico (Figure 15.9). The U.S. utilization includes both Texas and non-home-base states, where, as some respondents indicated, it is easier to access health care due to the less stringent Medicaid eligibility requirements and where the care is perceived to be better.

In the preceding 2-year period, 40% of the participants had visited a health provider 10 or more times, but a significant portion of these visits were for pediatric care. Approximately half of those interviewed sought medical attention from private physicians and clinics, and only 6% went to the hospitals for their medical needs (Figure 15.10). The almost exclusive use of private physicians by those who seek care in Mexico and by children insured through Medicaid accounts for the seemingly large number of migrant farmworker families who visit these health care providers.

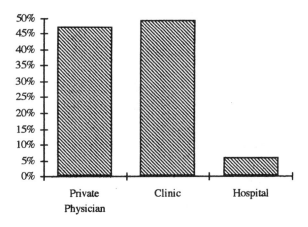

Figure 15.10. Providers Sought ($N = 47$)

The majority of the children born to the respondents were born in the United States. In both Mexico and the United States, the most common attendant at birth was a midwife. Fifty percent of the total births were delivered by lay midwives outside a formal medical facility, 36% were delivered in hospitals, and 14% were delivered in clinics (Figure 15.11). As was perceived and recalled by the respondents, the average cost for delivery was approximately $200 and $380 in Mexico and the United States, respectively.[3]

General Impressions

The population we surveyed was afflicted with many of the health and social problems that we had encountered in the literature. Inaccessibility to health care services, lack of transportation, and emphasis on curative as opposed to preventive care were common characteristics among the participants. Problems generally associated with low-income families were exacerbated when less common medical problems arose, as was the case with some of the participants.

Many of the farmworkers interviewed expressed concerns not only about their own health but about the health of others that they knew. One woman interviewed had a sister with an autoimmune skin disorder that required constant medical attention, but she was unable to receive care because she was uninsured and ineligible for Medicaid. Other participants

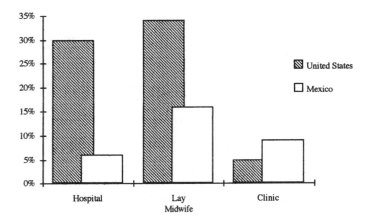

Figure 15.11. Country of Birth and Attendant at Delivery ($N = 210$)

indicated that the cost of medical services had inhibited them from seeking care. The shortage of doctors brings about a further concern that diseases will become too advanced before care can be sought.

A number of the participants stated that they were disappointed with the medical system in the United States. One reason for this is the farmworkers' perception that in the United States, the health care providers are more concerned with the insurance status of the patient than with the potential health problems. In Mexico, on the other hand, this concern is perceived to be the reverse, in that the Mexican providers are interested in addressing the patients' health problems before the patients' ability to pay. In addition, the farmworkers, especially those who were undocumented or had undocumented family members, often felt that they were being interrogated in the U.S. health care facilities, unlike facilities in Mexico.

We interviewed families who have children with disabilities, such as Down's syndrome, spina bifida, and a neurological disorder. The child with Down's was one of 11 children living with their parents in a mobile home with no hot water. Although half of the children were U.S. citizens (including the child with Down's), the mother stated that they had been chased away from clinics, where they were accused of "just wanting to use U.S. social services."

The child afflicted with spina bifida lived in a one-bedroom recreational trailer where six people were living. The parents slept in the back bedroom, and the four children shared a bed in the front area of the trailer.

At the time of the interview, the child was bathing in a tin washtub; the mother of the child stated that this was how she kept the child cool because there was no air conditioning and the ventilation in the trailer was poor.

Other comments concerned the feeling of alienation experienced by the farmworkers. The community health centers in Laredo and Brownsville are currently unable to accept new clients due to health provider shortages. Because these clinics receive MHP funding, the farmworkers feel that the clinics should be able to accommodate them, just as the clinics upstream do. The alienation felt is not only from the health care system in particular but from the area's population in general. The residents of Rio Bravo, located about 10 miles from Laredo, feel animosity from their neighbors in Laredo. For example, they have to travel to Highway 83 to receive emergency services because the ambulances will not enter the *colonia.*

Discussion

There were several limitations to this study. The sample size is small, and therefore the results cannot be assumed for the entire population of migrant and seasonal farmworkers. The size of the sample was affected by the fact that many farmworkers were in the migrant stream at the time of the interviews and by the disillusionment of many with surveys such as these. Farmworker advocates indicated that many farmworkers were frustrated when they participated in surveys and then saw no apparent improvements as a result.

There were some complications in the administration of interviews due to the lack of a direct translation from English to Spanish of some of the questions in the survey. The survey was written in English, but 45 of the 47 interviews were conducted in Spanish. Both authors are fluent in English and Spanish, but the inability to translate concepts unfamiliar to the respondents, such as preventive care, led to some difficulty in the translation.

The randomness of the sample was affected by the fact that some potential respondents were unwilling to talk to us without a community member present. The presence of the community member, although it allowed us to conduct the surveys, may have affected the way in which the participants responded.

Despite the limitations of the study, the impoverished conditions mentioned in much of the literature were evident in the population we surveyed (Wilk, 1986, p. 13). Interviews in Cameron Park were conducted during winter weather conditions, and aside from the need for general housing necessities previously mentioned, the lack of heat and proper insulation and the inferior housing materials—such that, for example, many homes had cracks in the walls—required that the inhabitants of the homes wear multiple layers of clothing to endure the cold. The unpaved roads and poor street drainage made it nearly impossible for residents to drive or walk when it rained.

A single mother with 10 children residing outside the Brownsville city limits lived in two dilapidated recreational trailers. The trailers had no plumbing hookup, and the family collected rainwater in outdoor barrels for drinking, cooking, and bathing. Much of the floor area was dirt covered, with decaying food and animal feces also strewn about. Social services had been unsuccessful in locating public housing for the family because of the occupancy limits per unit. When we went to interview the family, the children were unattended while the mother was in Mexico, and they had been relying on food found in the dumpsters of restaurants for their meals.

The general consensus of the participants was one of dissatisfaction with health care accessibility and services in the United States, especially in the home-base area. Complaints of the farmworkers interviewed included long lines to see providers, unavailability of immediate appointments, impersonal attention, and high cost of services due to lack of insurance and stringent Medicaid requirements. As a result of these problems, and as is consistent with the current literature, this population most commonly seeks curative rather than preventive health care services. Most migrant farmworkers interviewed also indicated that changes could be made to the current health care system, including the ability to pay for services through some sort of payment plan and a national health care program.

Areas for Further Research

The lack of research on migrant and seasonal farmworkers has combined with a lack of public policy that pertains to this population and a deficiency in other efforts that would prove advantageous to this population. One of the primary reasons for this deficiency is the problem of research and the methodology associated with that research. Much of the research done on migrant farmworkers is extremely out of date, having been done in the

1960s and 1970s (Arnold & Zuvekas, 1988, p. 2). More recently, census figures have been used in attempts at enumerating the farmworker population. The census data, however, are considered unreliable for this purpose because they are collected in April and categorize employment according to the job held most recently in the previous 2 weeks. Often, a migrant farmworker will not yet be performing agricultural work in April because the harvest seasons for many products have not yet arrived. Also, problems may arise because this population is undercounted in general and because the population home based in Mexico is missed entirely. Therefore, it is probable that a large portion of the migrant population is classified as being in some other employment or unemployed. Differences in definitions of what constitutes a migrant farmworker, as well as the inclusion or exclusion of dependents, are other potential difficulties in the attempts to count the farmworker population (National Advisory Council on Migrant Health, 1992, pp. 295-296).

The problems faced in enumerating the farmworker population accurately complicate the research of the health status of farmworkers. Some regional studies have been completed, but although these studies may be somewhat useful at the local, state, and possibly even stream levels, the applicability of these studies to the farmworker population as a whole is limited. Problems arise when, as often happens, these studies are used to represent the farmworker population at large. Often, when similar studies are conducted by separate agencies in different migrant streams, conflicting results are produced. The insufficient data on the population and on the study methodology itself make it difficult to determine which variables are producing the contradictory results. This is not to say, however, that it is impossible to obtain reliable health data for the farmworker population—only that a populationwide effort has not yet been made (Galarneau, 1992).

For the health status of the migrant and seasonal farmworker population to shift toward that of the general population, attention must be paid to these deficiencies, and changes must be made. These changes must be executed at all levels—from an increase in preventive services, health education, and outreach at the local migrant and community health center level, to the formulation of case management services and a viable data transfer system among the clinics in each stream and nationwide, all the way to the recognition of these problems in the nation's capital as legislation is formulated.

Because the migrant and seasonal farmworker population is so different from that of the United States in general, there is a need for a health care delivery system tailored to this population. This health care must be specific to their needs both as migrants and as a distinct culture (National Advisory Council on Migrant Health, 1993, p. 18). Preventive care, such as prenatal care for pregnant women, is a vital part of a health delivery system. Many of the migrant farmworker women fall into high-risk groups, have unplanned pregnancies, and are unable to afford care. The lack of prenatal care in the migrant farmworker population has led to an increased incidence of infant mortality, miscarriage, and pregnancy complications (National Advisory Council on Migrant Health, 1993, p. 37). Education of the farmworker population is another way of preventing some of the more basic health problems that they suffer. By training farmworkers in such essential concepts as nutrition, basic child care, recognition of symptoms of serious health difficulties, and the importance of timely attention to health problems, they will be better able to care for themselves and their families and will be more inclined to seek health care when they need it.

As previously mentioned, the farmworker population has a high need for medical attention, but the current funding for the migrant and community health centers is ineffective. The isolation of the workers and their frequent inability to reach the clinics have been cited as reasons for the extent to which health care is unavailable to farmworkers. Community outreach programs using both clinical and lay health advisors have proven effective in providing needed health care services to migrants. An increase in the number of these outreach programs, especially in the rural areas where federal clinics are nonexistent, will lead to improved health care for migrant and seasonal farmworkers nationwide (National Advisory Council on Migrant Health, 1993, p. 53).

An additional obstacle to serving migrant and seasonal farmworkers adequately is the inability to track individual workers and their health status. An information system would help diminish problems such as loss of medical records by the farmworkers and the inability to track the immunization status of children. Such a system would also be a necessary precedent to the much-needed viable data transfer system between clinics in a stream and nationwide (K. Mountain, personal communication, September 15, 1993). An electronic system that would allow the transfer of data from an upstream clinic to the patient's home-base clinic, providing the downstream clinic with information on the status of the patient and his or her treatment, would greatly decrease the duplication of treatments by different clinics. Because such a system will require both time and resources to develop, it is necessary to emphasize to farmworkers the importance of hand-carrying their medical records to the various health providers they seek in the stream.

Although the migrant and seasonal farmworker population is largely a minority population, traditional minority solutions are inadequate to treat their problems. The unique aspects of the migrant farmworker lifestyle require innovative and multicultural solutions. As one migrant farmworker stated, "Clinton said he would address health care; instead he has addressed wars in other countries. Meanwhile, we are fighting wars in our own country. The war against poverty, the war against poor health, the war against gangs, and the war against malnutrition. We are losing these wars."

Notes

1. For the purposes of this chapter, we will assume that all data refer to documented workers only, and we will refer only to this portion of the population.

2. For full site and client eligibility information, refer to Part D, Subpart I of Section 329 of the Public Health Service Act.

3. This does not include the cost of delivery and care of one child born prematurely, with a cerebral hemorrhage. The cost of this care was U.S. $415,000 (Arnold & Zuvekas, 1988).

References

Arnold, J., & Zuvekas, A. (1988). *Research agenda for community and migrant health centers.* Rockville, MD: U.S. Department of Health and Human Services.

Centers for Disease Control and Prevention. (1992). HIV infection, syphilis, and tuberculosis screening among migrant farm workers—Florida 1992. *Morbidity and Mortality Weekly Report, 41,* 723-725.

Dever, G. E. A. (1991). *Migrant health status: Profile of a population with complex health problems.* Austin, TX: Migrant Clinicians Network.

Foulk, D., Lafferty, J., Ryan, R., & Robertson, A. (1989). AIDS knowledge and risk behaviors of migrant and seasonal farmworkers in Georgia. *Migrant Health Newsline, 6*(4), 52-53.

Galarneau, C. A. (1992). Farmworkers as "different": A matter of difference or indifference? *Migration World Magazine, 20*(1), 29-33.

Goldfarb, R. L. (1981). *Migrant farmworkers: A caste of despair.* Ames: Iowa State University Press.

Hatcher, J., Hopewell, J., Guardiola, A., Jacquart, K., Moreau, W., Stys, J., DeNino, L., & Warner, D. (1995). *The Border Health Authority: Issues and design* (U.S.-Mexican Policy Studies Program Occasional Paper No. 6). Austin, TX: Lyndon B. Johnson School of Public Affairs.

Horton, D. G. (1989). Health care utilization by migrant farmworkers at their home base residences. *Migration World Magazine, 16*(3), 30-34.

Littlefield, C., & Stout, C. (1988, February/March). A survey of Colorado's migrant farmworkers: Access to health care. *Migrant Health Newsline, 5*(Suppl), 1-3.

Martin, P. L. (1988). *Harvest of confusion: Migrant workers in U.S. agriculture.* Boulder, CO: Westview.

Martin, P. L., & Taylor, J. E. (1988). *Harvest of confusion: SAWs, RAWs and farmworkers.* Washington, DC: Urban Institute.

Miller, N. L. (1990, November/December). Pullman Environmental Health Project. *Migrant Health Newsline, 7*(Suppl.), 97.

Mines, R., & Massey, D. S. (1985). Patterns of migration to the United States from two Mexican communities. *Latin American Research Review, 20,* 104-123.

National Advisory Council on Migrant Health. (1992). *Farmworker health for the year 2000: 1992 recommendations of the National Advisory Council on Migrant Health.* Austin, TX: National Migrant Resource Program.

National Advisory Council on Migrant Health. (1993). *1993 recommendations of the National Advisory Council on Migrant Health.* Rockville, MD: Author.

National Association of Community Health Centers, Inc. (1991). *Medicaid and migrant farmworker families: Analysis of barriers and recommendations for change.* Washington, DC: Author.

National Association of Community Health Centers, Inc. (1996). *21st Annual Policy and Issues Forum: Forging a new consensus: What health centers must do next.* Washington, DC: Author.

National Migrant Resource Program, Inc. (n.d.). *Fact sheet: Basic health.* Austin, TX: Author.

National Migrant Resource Program, Inc. (1990a). *Migrant and seasonal farmworker health objectives for the year 2000.* Austin, TX: Author.

National Migrant Resource Program, Inc. (1990b). *1990 migrant health centers referral directory.* Austin, TX: Author.

Plascencia, L. F. B., Ceballos, M., & Glover, R. W. (1989). *Texas Farmworker Enumeration Project: A report prepared for the National Migrant Referral Project.* Austin, TX: Center for the Study of Human Resources, Lyndon B. Johnson School of Public Affairs.

Robinson, J. (1990, January/February). The Camp Health Aide Program. *Migrant Health Newsline, 7*(Suppl.), 69.

Rust, G. (1990). Health status of migrant farmworkers: A literature review and commentary. *American Journal of Public Health, 80,* 1213-1217.

Sakala, C. (1987). Migrant and seasonal farmworkers in the United States: A review of health hazards, status and policy. *International Migration Review, 21,* 659-687.

Stoddard, E. (1984). Northern Mexican migration and the U.S./Mexico border region. *New Scholar, 9,*(1-2), 51-72.

Warner, D. (1991). Health issues at the U.S.-Mexican border. *Journal of the American Medical Association, 265,* 242-247.

Wilk, V. (1986). *The occupational health of migrant and seasonal farmworkers in the United States.* Washington, DC: Farmworker Justice Fund, Inc.

Wright, G. (1993). *Feasibility study to develop a Medicaid reciprocity program for migrant and seasonal farmworkers: Background paper.* (Available from the Health Care Finance Administration, Baltimore, MD 21244).

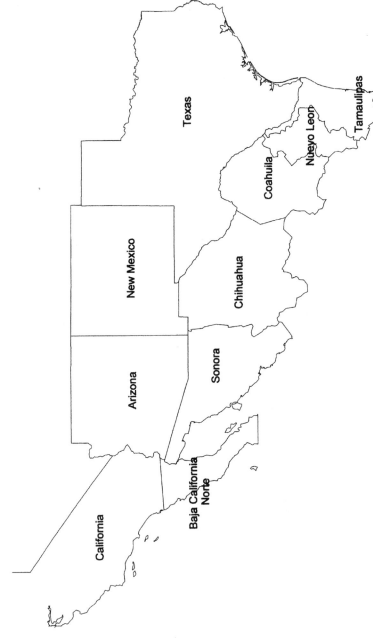

Appendix A. Map of the U.S.-Mexico Border Region

Appendix B

Example of an Exercise From the Curriculum Used During Intervention A

LIST OF "A JOB WELL DONE"

If you are ready for a regular job, it would be a good idea to evaluate each potential job situation to see how well you could fill the requirements of recuperation. The following questions can help you to evaluate the job. Of course, no job is perfect, and some of the questions cannot be answered completely. For example, if you have already begun to work, some of the questions are not relevant.

It would be very useful for you to try to answer these questions as completely and honestly as possible before accepting a job offer. Each negative answer ("no") suggests a need for you to take on and resolve the point discussed. Some "no" answers may show that even though job opportunities are scarce, the one you are looking at is not appropriate for you.

1. Does this offer you the salary you presently need?
2. Will you have adequate transportation?
3. Do you have a clear idea of what this job will entail?
4. Do you now have or think you could soon acquire the abilities needed for this job?
5. Is the atmosphere at work safe and reasonably pleasant?
6. Will the job be permanent and for the whole year? Will you be paid regularly?
7. Does this job include adequate supervision and evaluations that will help you in your work?
8. Will the job offer opportunities to improve your abilities and/or offer advancement?
9. Do you feel that this job is challenging?
10. Will the work environment be free from situations, places, and people that have strongly tempted you to consume drugs in the past?

Appendix C

Example of a Discussion Exercise From the Curriculum Used During Intervention B

HAVING FUN WITHOUT DRUGS

We all have the need to have pleasurable moments, and quitting drugs should not mean that we are also quitting the fun times. In fact, a person whose mind, body, and lifestyle have no more addictions can have fun in many different ways, but we must learn to have fun without drugs.

The majority of pleasures that do not include drugs, however, do involve some physical activity. A person who has depended on drugs to have fun and whose nervous system is used to artificial stimulation must readjust to this new drug-free reality. The question is then: What do you need to learn and do to have fun and feel satisfied without using drugs?

You need to be smart to have fun without drugs.

- **Participation**—You should participate in the activities we will be providing from time to time. You should try to do this on a regular basis until they become a habit.

- **Enthusiasm**—Try to reflect on everything you do. You don't need to jump for joy all the time, but at least be willing to enjoy yourself. Don't fall back on your old prejudices and say, "This is not for me," or "I never liked this before." Remember that you are changing. Your attitudes and expectations have a lot to do with how you will experience new things.

- **Practice**—Enjoying new things is part of a process. You must try out new things, increase your confidence in your abilities, and continue doing those things you enjoy the most as part of your lifestyle. It takes time, but the pleasures experienced without drugs increase with time and practice.

- **Support**—It is difficult for lonely people to feel well. It is much easier to feel well when one has many friends. And what your friends like to do has a great influence on what you like to do. Find new friends, and establish your priorities so you may share the good moments with them without having to use drugs.

Appendix D

Survey of Migrant Farmworkers in South Texas

1. Sex: M F
2. Age: _____
3. Are you married?
   a. yes
   b. no
4. Do you have children living with you?
   a. yes (how many and ages)
   b. no
5. Do the children go to school (if they are school aged)?
   a. yes (where?)
   b. no
6. Do you own or rent your house?
   a. own
   b. rent
7. How many people are living in your house?
   a. 1-3
   b. 4-6
   c. 7-9
   d. 10 or more
8. How many bedrooms are in your house?
   a. 0
   b. 1
   c. 2
   d. 3 or more
9. Does your home have running water? indoor plumbing? electricity?
   a. yes   a. yes   a. yes
   b. no   b. no   b. no
10. Are you eligible for food stamps?
    a. yes
    b. no

11. If yes, do you receive food stamps?
    a. yes
    b. no

12. Do you leave the area to obtain farmwork (migratory), or do you do farmwork only in this area (seasonal)?
    a. migratory
    b. seasonal (go to Questions #16-18, then to #22)

13. Do you migrate out of Texas?
    a. yes (to what states?)
    b. no

14. What is the duration of your migration (per year)?
    a. 0-2 months
    b. 3-4 months
    c. 5-6 months
    d. 7-8 months
    e. 9-10 months
    f. 11-12 months

15. When did you enter the migrant stream?
    a. 0-1 year ago
    b. 1-3 years ago
    c. 3-5 years ago
    d. more than 5 years ago

16. Where are you originally from?
    a. United States (what state?)
    b. Mexico (what state?)

17. Do you have relatives in Mexico?
    a. yes (what states?)
    b. no

18. How long have been living in the U.S.?
    a. 0-1 year
    b. 1-3 years
    c. 3-5 years
    d. more than 5 years

19. How long have you been living in this home base area?
    a. 0-1 year
    b. 1-3 years
    c. 3-5 years
    d. more than 5 years

20. When you travel, who do you travel with? (circle all that apply)
    a. alone
    b. with spouse
    c. with children
    d. with other extended family members
    e. with others (friends/neighbors/etc.)

21. If you are traveling with family members, do any of them work? (circle all that apply)
    a. none
    b. all
    c. spouse
    d. child(ren)
    e. other extended family members

22. When you are ill, do you seek medical attention?
    a. yes
    b. no (why not?) (go to Question #25)

23. Do you go to: (circle all that apply)
    a. private physician
    b. clinic
    c. hospital
    e. other

24. Where do you seek medical attention?
    a. U.S. (for migratory, what state and facility)
    b. Mexico

25. Under what circumstances do you think medical care should be sought? (circle all that apply)
    a. routine checkup (i.e., prenatal, annual physical, etc.)
    b. acute illness (i.e., ear infection, bladder infection, pesticide exposure, etc.)
    c. chronic illness (i.e., diabetes, hypertension, etc.)
    d. muscular pain/discomfort
    e. other

26. Under what circumstances do you actually seek medical attention? (circle all that apply)
    a. routine checkup (i.e., prenatal, annual physical, etc.)
    b. acute illness (i.e., ear infection, bladder infection, pesticide exposure, etc.)
    c. chronic illness (i.e., diabetes, hypertension, etc.)

    d. muscular pain/discomfort

    e. other

27. What medical services do you know of that are available to you?

    a. private physician

    b. clinic

    c. hospital

    d. other

28. What type of medical insurance do you have?

    a. none (see Question #29)

    b. Medicaid

    c. Medicare

    d. private

    e. other

29. If no insurance, why not?

    a. ineligible

    b. can't afford

    c. don't want

    d. uniformed as to how to obtain

30. What medical problems have you had in the past two years?

    a. routine checkup (i.e., prenatal, annual physical, etc.)

    b. acute illness (i.e., ear infection, bladder infection, pesticide exposure, etc.)

    c. chronic illness (i.e., diabetes, hypertension, etc.)

    d. muscular pain/discomfort

    e. other

31. Did you seek medical attention?

    a. yes

    b. no

32. If yes, how much were you charged for the services?

    a. no charge

    b. insurance paid in full?

    c. $0-$50

    d. $51-$100

    e. $101-$250

    f. greater than $250

33. How many times in the past two years have you visited a health care provider?

    a. 0

    b. 1-3

    c. 4-6

    d. 7-9

    e. 10 or more

34. How much have you paid out of pocket for medical care in the past year?

    a. $0-$50

    b. $51-$200

    c. $201-$400

    d. greater than $400

35. Where were your children born?

    a. United States (what state/facility?)

    b. Mexico (what state?)

36. Were you charged for this?

    a. yes (how much?)

    b. no

37. Did you receive prenatal care?

    a. yes (where?)

    b. no

38. What problems do you see with medical care presently?

39. What concerns do you have about medical care?

40. What possible improvements do you think are necessary?

41. Are you aware of others who have medical problems that are not being taken care of?

INDEX

ABOUT THE CONTRIBUTORS

Michael D. Barnes, PhD, CHES, is Associate Professor of Health Science at Brigham Young University and holds a doctorate in community health education from Southern Illinois University in Carbondale. His current research and grant activities include strategic planning and assessment of *promotora* programs, media advocacy campaigns, and stress-coping assessments and interventions.

Sandra Benavides-Vaello was educated at the University of Texas at Austin, where she received a BSc in Nursing and an MA in public affairs from the Lyndon Baines Johnson School of Public Affairs. She is currently pursuing doctoral studies in nursing, also at the University of Texas at Austin. She is employed as Director of Clinical Affairs for the Texas Association of Community Health Centers, a private nonprofit health organization. Her research interests include health accessibility issues for high-risk populations, health issues for Mexican American women of low socioeconomic status, maternal and child health issues, and health concerns of migrant and seasonal farmworkers.

Theresa Byrd has spent most of her career working with U.S.-Mexico border and migrant populations, first in Arizona and then in California, Texas, and Chihuahua. As a public health nurse, she became aware of the special problems of low-income, marginalized populations, including the difficulties they have accessing the health care system. After receiving her MPH from the University of California at Los Angeles, she worked with *colonia* residents in Ciudad Juárez, Chihuahua, and El Paso, Texas, assisting in community development and health efforts. She has also been involved for several years with an organization dedicated to bringing appropriate technology water systems to the *ejidos* near Reynosa, Tamaulipas. After completing her DrPH at the University of Texas (UT)-Houston School of Public Health, she returned to El Paso as faculty for the UT-Houston School of Public Health satellite campus. Her research interests include border health issues, maternal and child health, community organizing, and perceptions of risk.

Robbin D. Crabtree received her MA and PhD in speech communication from the University of Minnesota (in 1987 and 1992, respectively). She is now Assistant Professor of Communication Studies at New Mexico State University, where she teaches courses in international, intercultural, and development communication as well as qualitative research methods. She has conducted research in Nicaragua, El Salvador, Cuba, India, and Kenya and along the U.S.-Mexico border, with a particular interest in participatory and action research methods.

Graciela De la Rosa is a social psychologist and was formerly Professor of Sociology at the Autonomous Metropolitan University in Mexico City. She is currently Research Coordinator for the Mexican Federation for Private Associations for Community Development (FEMAP) and is coordinating HIV/AIDS prevention programs for factory workers and female sex workers.

Jo Fairbanks has a PhD in community health education and more than 20 years of experience as a public health practitioner. She is currently coauthoring a textbook in public health and is teaching in the graduate program in public health at the University of New Mexico. Her areas of interest include rural health and public health policy. She has conducted research in nursing employment trends in New Mexico and in the use of community health workers as change agents in rural communities.

João B. Ferreira-Pinto, PhD (University of California at Irvine), is Assistant Professor of Behavioral Sciences at the University of Texas at Houston School of Public Health. His main research interests are in the area of HIV/AIDS prevention, especially as it relates to drug use. He is currently working on the cultural factors involved in the decision-making process of drug use initiation and cessation among injecting drug users in the United States and in Mexico.

Leigh Arden Ford is Assistant Professor of Communication Studies at New Mexico State University and holds a doctorate in organizational communication from Purdue University. She teaches upper division and graduate courses in organizational communication and in health communication. Her research interests emphasize the communication of social support and the communication of persuasive health-related messages. Current research activities include an interdisciplinary, granted project in cooperation with the Centers for Disease Control and Prevention and the New Mexico Department of Health assessing Spanish-language hantavirus prevention materials, an interdisciplinary project assessment of *promotoras* programs, and projects focused on the communication of social support among nurses and the communication practices of emergency department personnel. She has published articles in *Health Communication, Communication Monographs,* and *Communication Quarterly* and has made several presentations at national and regional conferences.

Irma Hinojosa started working in the transplant field in 1992. She brought her background in marketing (hotel, banking, and hospital) and public relations to a field previously exclusive to health care professionals. Her goal at Southwest Transplant Alliance was to increase consent rates for donation, especially among Hispanics, by improving the interaction with grieving families and developing programs with hospital staff key to the donation process. She studied English literature at the University of Texas at El Paso and the University of California at Los Angeles. She is a member of the Texas Alliance for Healthcare Marketing and Public Relations, the American Society for Health and Transplant Professionals, and the North American Transplant Coordinators Organization and has spoken on the subject of increasing minority consent rate at national conferences for both the American Society for Health and Transplant Professionals and the North American Transplant Coordinators Organization. She is also an accredited bereavement facilitator.

Jillian Hopewell is the Director of Education and Professional Development for the Migrant Clinicians Network in Austin, Texas. She holds an MA in Latin American studies and an MA in public administration from the University of Texas at Austin.

Michael P. Kelly, PhD (Texas A&M University), is a Certified Health Education Specialist. He is currently Assistant Professor in the Health Science Program at the University of Texas at El Paso. In addition to his current work on diabetes screening and education with Roman Catholic churches along the Texas-Mexico border, he is involved in research pertaining to integration of health education programming into Christian youth activities and organizing interfaith care for the sick in the border region.

Jesusa Lara (EdD, RN) is Associate Professor in the College of Nursing and Health Sciences, University of Texas at El Paso. She is currently Education Director of the Kellogg Community Partnerships Project for the college. She was previously Project Director of the School Centered Health Education and Services for Rural Communities from 1990 to 1993, funded by the W. K. Kellogg Foundation.

Patricia A. Lawrence (PhD, 1990, University of Kentucky) taught theory and research methods and was Graduate Advisor in the Department of Communication at the University of Texas at El Paso when she conducted the research for this book chapter. She also was Principal Investigator on a grant from the National Science Foundation. Much of her published research focuses on the effects of sensation- and novelty-seeking needs on illicit substance use and on mass media consumption. She currently teaches in the School of Communication at the University of Idaho. She has been active in public health projects in a number of Latin American countries, including Ecuador, Mexico, Peru, Paraguay, and the Dominican Republic.

Sheila Murphy received her PhD in social psychology in 1990 from the University of Michigan. Since that time, she has been a full-time faculty member at the Annenberg School for Communication at the University of Southern California (USC). Her research interests focus on the impact of various factors such as ethnicity and emotion in decision making. Over the past several years, she has received federal funding to study such diverse topics as the role of ethnicity in end-of-life decisions, individuals' perceptions of their ethical and legal obligations to undergo genetic testing, and the decision to engage in unprotected sex among populations at high risk for contracting HIV. In addition to being an Associate Professor at USC, she is a consultant for the Centers for Disease Control and Prevention in Atlanta.

Ellen M. Parietti received a BS from Emory University in 1990 with a dual major in biological anthropology and ecology. She served as a Peace Corps volunteer in Costa Rica from 1991 to 1993, working in reforestation. On her return, she enrolled in the University of Texas at Houston School of Public Health's El Paso campus. She completed her MPH in 1995. While completing her public health degree, she worked in El Paso's public health clinics and volunteered with the area's farmworker organization. As a result of her work with the immigrant community in El Paso, she developed an understanding of the area of women's health issues and health problems of Hispanic childbearing women. She continues to work in the field of international health and is currently employed by the International Eye Foundation as a Program Officer for Latin America, working in the prevention of blindness in developing countries.

J. Gerard Power (PhD, Annenberg School for Communication, University of Southern California) is a Senior Research Analyst with Frank N. Magid Associates Inc., New York City. He has lived and worked in Mexico and on the U.S.-Mexico border. His research interests include adolescent health promotion, media and identity, and the use of counterstereotypes to reduce prejudice. His work has been published in the *Journal of Health Communication, Communication Research,* the *Journal of Communication Inquiry,* and *Human Communication Research.*

Jesus Ramirez-Valles is Assistant Professor of Community Health Sciences in the University of Illinois-Chicago School of Public Health. He received his MPH and PhD in health education from the University of Michigan. His research interests include the sociology of health promotion, community-based health education, gender, race, and HIV/AIDS.

Maria E. Ramos has a BS in social work from the Autonomous University of Ciudad Juárez and is currently completing a master's thesis on the history of drug use in Juárez since the 1900s. As Director of the Drug Abuse Program for Compañeros, she has played a central role in the research initiatives of the National Institute of Drug Abuse and the Center for Substance Abuse Prevention.

Rebeca L. Ramos, MA, MPH, is the Executive Director of Compañeros HIV/AIDS and Heroin Treatment Programs and the Principal Investigator on an HIV/STD Training and Technical Assistance Grant for the U.S.-Mexico border region provided by the Centers for Disease Control and

Prevention. She serves as a consultant with a number of national and international government agencies and private organizations in the United States and Latin America and has served as an advisor for both the United States and Mexico on presidential task forces concerning HIV issues.

Bill Schlesinger is Codirector, with Carol Schlesinger, of Project Vida, a community-based multiple service social agency in El Paso, Texas, that was selected as a 1996 winner in the "Models That Work" campaign, cosponsored by the federal Health Resources and Services Administration (HRSA) along with many other national agencies. He is an ordained Presbyterian minister and an adjunct faculty member of McCormick Theological Seminary's Doctor of Ministry program.

Heather Setzler holds a BSc in Spanish from Pacific University in Forest Grove, Oregon, and an MA in Latin American studies from the University of Texas at Austin. She currently works as Project Coordinator at the IC2 Institute, a technology think tank and research consortium at the University of Texas at Austin. Her research interests include health care accessibility issues in the United States and Latin America, disadvantaged populations, and migration issues.

Enrique Suarez, MD, is Director of the Mexican Federation of Private Associations for Community Development (FEMAP). He has conducted several research projects on child and mental health, drug abuse prevention, and community health education.

Marc A. Zimmerman, PhD, is an Associate Professor in the Department of Health Behavior and Health Education in the School of Public Health and in the Combined Program in Education and Psychology at the University of Michigan. He is also the editor of *Health Education and Behavior.* He received his PhD in psychology from the University of Illinois. His research interests include application and development of empowerment theory, the study of adolescent health and resiliency, and HIV/AIDS prevention.